Health Disparities and the Ancestral Environment

Health Disparities and the Ancestral Environment:

An Evolutionary Perspective

By

Anthony R. Mawson

Cambridge Scholars Publishing

Health Disparities and the Ancestral Environment:
An Evolutionary Perspective

By Anthony R. Mawson

This book first published 2023

Cambridge Scholars Publishing

Lady Stephenson Library, Newcastle upon Tyne, NE6 2PA, UK

British Library Cataloguing in Publication Data
A catalogue record for this book is available from the British Library

ISBN (10): 1-5275-1466-8
ISBN (13): 978-1-5275-1466-9

TABLE OF CONTENTS

Other Essays

PREFACE

For nearly two decades I was honored to be a professor of epidemiology and biostatistics in the School of Public Health at Jackson State University, an historically black college and university (HBCU). During the years 2006-2010 I was a professor of pediatrics and medicine at the University of Mississippi Medical Center. There I began teaching a graduate school course of health disparities. I was also honored to serve as the first principal investigator of the National Children's Study for Mississippi.

In earlier years at Jackson State University, I helped to organize several national conferences on eliminating health disparities, and two annual training courses on research career survival skills for junior minority faculty. Development of these training courses was in partnership with the University of Pittsburg's Center for Minority Health. I returned to JSU in 2011 with an investigator-initiated research grant from Pfizer. The research aimed to test a hypothesis on the role of retinoids in onchocerciasis, and it involved a partnership with colleagues at the Tanzanian Institute for Medical Research. I continued to teach a graduate course on health disparities and participated in helping to prepare JSU to become, in 2018, the first accredited School of Public Health at an HBCU in the nation.

These and other experiences deepened my knowledge and curiosity about health disparities affecting African Americans. The theory proposed here also derives partly from my long-standing research interest in the role of vitamin A in health and disease, which began as a graduate student at Tulane University's School of Public Health and Tropical Medicine. Vitamin A is considered an essential nutrient, as the term "vitamin" implies. However, increasing evidence implicates it contributing to the causation of many chronic diseases and to certain acute infectious diseases, associated with reduced risks in people of African descent; that is, health disparities in the "reverse" direction.

During their life cycle, malaria parasites spend over a week in the liver, where over 90% of vitamin A in the body is stored. Malaria parasites selectively absorb vitamin A from the human host, and people of sub-Saharan African descent are at reduced risk of severe malaria compared to people of European descent. In 2013 I proposed the hypothesis that, upon emerging from the liver the merozoite-stage parasites, packed with vitamin A, use it as a membrane destabilizer to invade and reproduce in the red blood cells. On the death of these cells in very large numbers the vitamin A is released into the circulation in toxic concentrations, inducing the signs and symptoms of the disease. This hypothesis was supported by a study published in 2019.[1] The study confirmed previous findings of low serum retinol in patients with malaria. However, it also reported for the first time that concentrations of retinoic acid, the major biologically active and potentially toxic metabolite of vitamin A, were significantly increased.

How are people of sub-Saharan Africa protected against death from malaria? The foregoing led me to conceive the idea that this protection has resulted from physiological adaptations to the impact of endemic malaria parasitism, related to vitamin A, evolving over the course of millennia. The hypothesized adaptations included: 1) sequestering vitamin A away from the liver to other organs, thereby reducing access to its use by the invaders in causing disease; and 2) slowing the metabolism and breakdown of vitamin A, causing it to accumulate in the body to sub-toxic levels that weakened the parasites and thereby reduced the risk of severe disease.

These adaptations may have served to protect against severe malaria and some other diseases in the ancestral environment. However, they may also have simultaneously increased risks of chronic diseases for people of West Central African descent exposed to the typical dairy-based US diet, which is high in preformed vitamin A. These adaptations are hypothesized to increase susceptibility to chronic inflammatory diseases in which retinoids may play a causative role, notably atopy, vascular diseases, diabetes, and cancer, as well as genetic diseases such as sickle cell anemia and glucose-6-phosphate dehydrogenase deficiency. In short, the same physiological adaptations that are protective against tropical diseases, coupled with exposure to a dairy-based diet, may be contributing to persisting health differences in African Americans.

References

1. Na J, Khan A, Kim JK, Wadood A, Choe YL, Walker DI, Jones DP, Lim CS, Park YH. Discovery of metabolic alterations in the serum of patients infected with Plasmodium spp. by high-resolution metabolomics. Metabolomics. 2019 Dec 23;16(1):9. doi: 10.1007/s11306-019-1630-2. PMID: 31872321.

ACKNOWLEDGMENTS

I wish to thank my scientific collaborators and former colleagues Drs. Ashley Croft, Azad Bhuiyan, Federico Gonzalez-Fernandez, Suvankar Majumdar, and Amal Mitra for the opportunity to collaborate with them on research that has led to several publications on or involving infectious diseases, cancer, neurodevelopmental disorders, and vitamin A. I am also grateful to Dr. Marinelle Payton, Professor and Chair of JSU's Department of Epidemiology and Biostatistics, for her collegiality and support of my research at Jackson State University.

I also thank my graduate students in public health at Jackson State University, among whom Juliet Enow, Veronica Hernandez, and Kendrick Walker in particular provided valuable critical comments and help in gathering data for this essay on health disparities; and also Robyn Howard, for preparing the graphics.

I am especially grateful to Dr. Omar Bagasra, whom I met at a conference on zika, for inviting me to present an early version of the proposed theory of health disparities at the South Carolina Center for Biotechnology, Claflin University, in March 2017. I also thank participants in the Distinguished Seminar Series, Research Centers in Minority Institutions and Center for Environmental Health (RCMI-CEH), Jackson State University, March 29, 2017, for their valuable critical comments on my presentation, "Toward a theory of health disparities affecting people of sub-Saharan African descent."

Finally, I thank my wife Carol Andersen for preparing the Index, for her editorial skills and overall support, and for our two lovely daughters since 2001. My sister Lucy Kinna, also kindly assisted in editing the manuscript for publication.

CHAPTER ONE

GENERAL INTRODUCTION

Human populations have adapted to diverse aspects of their environment, such as climate and pathogens, leaving signatures of genetic variation.[1,2] This well-established principle may apply to African Americans – people of mainly West Central African descent – who are at increased risk of many vascular, metabolic, malignant, and allergic diseases compared to their European counterparts. In 2021 there were an estimated 40.1 million people self-identifying as non-Hispanic black or African American, representing 12.1 percent of the total United States population of 331.9 million. Blacks/African Americans are the second largest minority population in the United States, after the Hispanic/Latino population. Concentrated primarily in the southern states, African Americans are projected to comprise 15% (60.7 million) by 2060.[3]

The prevailing view of health disparities affecting African Americans – inequities in health care access, quality, and health outcomes – is that they result from many factors, particularly social, economic and environmental. Racial inequities are estimated to cost the nation a total of $135 billion per year, including $93 billion in excess medical costs and $42 billion in lost productivity.[4] Disproportionately poor health outcomes – in infant mortality, life expectancy and the prevalence of chronic disease—reveal differences by race and ethnicity, independent of other factors, that are widely attributed to health system, educational, residential, and other forms of discrimination.[5]

> "In the past few years, amid a pandemic [COVID-19] that has taken a disproportionate toll on Black and brown people and a national reckoning on racial justice, leaders from several U.S. health systems have named racism as a public health threat and pledged to identify and reverse racist policies and practices in their institutions. As an example, in an open letter published last Juneteenth, leaders from 36 Chicago hospitals said it's 'time for action' and promised to 'double down' on efforts to reduce racial health disparities among their patients, create more equitable workplaces for their employees, and invest in communities of color where many of their patients and staff live ... In several institutions, this work has been spurred by medical students or residents demanding change." [6]

Certain observations on the health of African Americans across the age span are not readily explained by structural racism, discrimination, or other social factors. For instance, it is not widely known that people originally from sub-Saharan Africa are at reduced risk of death from other diseases, notably malaria, dengue hemorrhagic fever, yellow fever, and nonalcoholic fatty liver disease. These mostly infectious diseases are prevalent in tropical West Central Africa, suggesting genetic links between the natural environment and endemic disease and hinting at a role for nonsocial factors in the explanation of health disparities.

Here the case is made that disparities in *health outcomes* affecting African Americans are partly the result of physiological adaptations to the vectors of major infectious diseases in the ancestral environment of sub-Saharan Africa, occurring on an evolutionary timescale, coupled with the impact of the natural and dairy-based nutritional environment of North America. The sub-Saharan African environment has involved continuous exposure to potentially lethal tropical diseases, a major one being *Plasmodium falciparum* malaria, the most dangerous form of the disease. Together with other parasitic organisms, *Plasmodium falciparum* selectively absorbs vitamin A from the human host and uses it in reproduction and disease pathogenesis.

Vitamin A is a major constituent of the dairy-and egg-based diet of North America. Less well known is that vitamin A is a potentially toxic fat-soluble molecule that is stored mainly in the liver as retinyl esters, and it contributes importantly to many acute and chronic conditions and diseases, including parasitic diseases and diabetes.

On the proposed theory, inherited physiological characteristics acquired over millennia from evolutionary adaptations to endemic tropical diseases – including malaria, schistosomiasis, and onchocerciasis – render people of West Central African descent particularly sensitive to vitamin A as a toxin. The proposed evolutionary adaptations were 1) sequestering vitamin A away from the liver, where it is mainly stored, to other organs, to reduce accessibility to *Plasmodia*; and 2) slowing the metabolism and catabolism of vitamin A, causing it to accumulate to subtoxic concentration, thereby weakening the parasite and serving to reduce the risk of severe disease.

These adaptations may have helped to enhance survival in the original African environment. However, in the North American environment, characterized by the absence of vitamin A-absorbing parasites and by a dairy-based diet that is rich in vitamin A, derived from the historic dependence of people of northern European descent on grazing animals, these adaptations are hypothesized to cause vitamin A to accumulate, rendering people of West Central African descent sensitive to vitamin A as a cellular toxin and at greater risk of the same chronic diseases that affect European Americans. The increased concentration of vitamin A in organs outside the liver, coupled with its excess overall accumulation, are proposed to explain the susceptibility of African Americans to organ-specific diseases that were once rare in the original environment and are increasingly linked to vitamin A toxicity via mitochondrial dysfunction and apoptosis.

On this theory, people of West Central African descent are more sensitive to vitamin A as a toxin than people of European descent, and disparities in chronic diseases are partly due to excess expression of the same retinoid-related mechanisms that are responsible for these diseases in general. Among its testable implications, the vitamin A toxicity hypothesis suggests that adoption of traditional or modified West Central African-style diets that are low in vitamin A and high in vitamin A-absorbing fiber could help to prevent and treat these diseases. Subject to testing, they could also serve as a population-based strategy for maintaining overall health and increasing longevity.

References

1. Omenn GS. Evolution in health and medicine Sackler colloquium: Evolution and public health. Proc Natl Acad Sci U S A. 2010 Jan 26;107 Suppl 1(Suppl 1):1702-9. doi: 10.1073/pnas.0906198106. Epub 2009 Dec 4.
2. James WPT, Johnson RJ, Speakman JR, et al. Nutrition and its role in human evolution. J Intern Med 2019; May;285(5):533-549. doi: 10.1111/joim.12878. Epub 2019 Feb 17.)
3. US Census Bureau. PEPSR6H-Annual Estimates of the Resident Population by Sex, Race, and Hispanic Origin for the United States, States, and Counties: April 1, 2010 to July 1, 2017.
4. W.K. Kellogg Foundation. The Business Case for Racial Equity: A Strategy for Growth. 2018. https://altarum.org/sites/default/files/uploaded-publication-files/WKKellogg_Business-Case-RacialEquity_National-Report_2018.pdf. (Accessed December 13, 2022).
5. NCSL National Conference of State Legislatures. Health Disparities Overview. https://www.ncsl.org/research/health/health-disparities-overview.aspx (Accessed December 13, 2022).
6. The Commonwealth Fund. Martha Hostetter and Sarah Klein, “Confronting Racism in Health Care: Moving from Proclamations to

New Practices," feature article, Commonwealth Fund, Oct. 18, 2021. https://doi.org/10.26099/kn6g-aa68. (Accessed December 14, 2022).

CHAPTER TWO

HEALTH DISPARITIES AFFECTING AFRICAN AMERICANS

An estimated 44 million Americans of African ancestry are now living in the United States, mostly from forced relocation over preceding centuries. The countries of origin were in West and Central Africa and included the Congo and Angola (39%), Togo, Benin, and Western Nigeria (20%), East Nigeria (15%), and the Cameroons, Equatorial Guinea, and Gabon (15%).[1] (Figure 1). For reasons that are not fully understood, African Americans, comprising 13% of the US population, are at greater risk of disease and/or death than Americans of European descent from the following:

- Cancers of the blood and bone marrow, breast, lung, ovary, prostate, colon, and rectum;[2,3]
- Metabolic and cardiovascular diseases including hypertension, type 2 diabetes, kidney disease, obesity, gout, congestive heart failure, and stroke;[4,5]
- Eczema;[6-8] asthma;[9] and allergies to eggs and milk.[10,11]

These conditions were once rare in African countries themselves.[12] Yet today the prevalence of hypertension in African Americans is over 40%, which is among the highest in the world. It also occurs earlier in life and is of greater severity than among other groups.[13] African Americans are also at risk of certain genetic diseases and conditions that include sickle cell anemia – the most common blood disorder in the US – and glucose-6-phosphate dehydrogenase deficiency (G6PDd), which is found almost exclusively among males from malaria-endemic regions.[14]

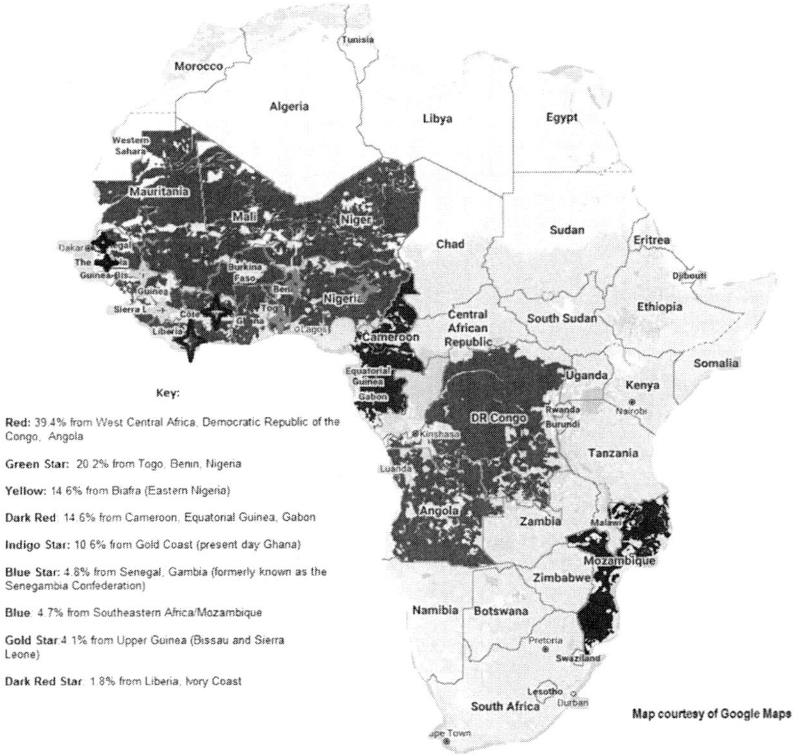

Figure 1. Ancestral origins of African Americans

Life expectancy is also shorter for African Americans compared to European Americans. Although it increased for both males and females from 1980–2014, it was 6.9 years longer for European American than for African American males and 5.6 years longer for European American females than for African American females.[15]

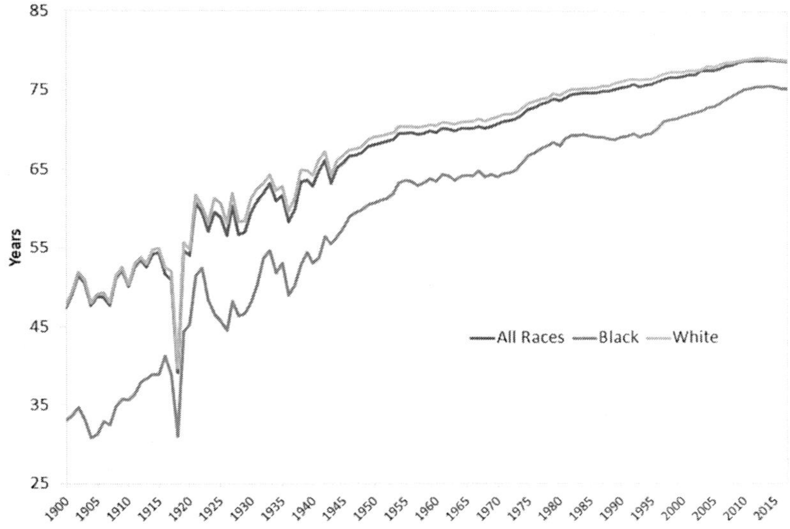

FEDERAL RESERVE BANK OF ST. LOUIS
https://www.stlouisfed.org/on-the-economy/2022/january/evolution-racial-gap-us-life-expectancy
SOURCES: NCHS, National Vital Statistics System and authors' calculations.
NOTES: Data end in 2017. For 1900 to 1969, Black life expectancy is based on data for the nonwhite population. From 1970 onward, the Black life expectancy is based on data for the Black or African American population. Both white and Black definitions include people of Hispanic and non-Hispanic origin.

The infant mortality rate for African American infants (deaths in infants up to 12 months of age per 1,000 live births) is more than twice that of European American infants, due to higher rates of stillbirth, birth defects, low birth weight, premature birth, and Sudden Infant Death Syndrome.[16-18] Rates of maternal mortality among African Americans are also close to three times higher than those of women of European descent.[19]

Infant gestational age, an important predictor of death and illness in infants, differs among racial and ethnic groups. Among the five groups measured in the National Vital Statistics Survey (NVSS) in 2014, African American women had the highest percentage of preterm singleton births at 11.1 percent, while Asian or Pacific Islander women had the lowest at 6.8 percent (NCHS, 2016).[20]

Death rates from cancer, diabetes and heart disease in sub-Saharan Africa are expected to exceed those from infectious diseases by 2030. As many as 46% of Africans suffer from high blood pressure, the highest rate worldwide, and a growing percentage of people are overweight.[21] Even in the mid-1990s the prevalence of diabetes exceeded that of the white population in Durban, South Africa.[22] Yet less than a century earlier coronary heart disease was rare in many parts of Africa,[23] as it was in western populations before World War I.[24] Cancer rates in Africa were also low.[25]

Changes in diet may have contributed to these statistics. Many countries in sub-Saharan Africa are adopting 'western' diets and are experiencing high rates of overweight and death from chronic diseases.[26]

References

1. Lima CAF. Tracing the genetic origin of African descendants from South America. Biol Anthropol Doctoral Thesis (2015). Retrieved from: https://tel.archives-ouvertes.fr/tel-01379619/document (Accessed November 1, 2020).
2. Long B, Liu F, Bristow R. Disparities in uterine cancer epidemiology, treatment, and survival among African Americans in the United States. Gynecol Oncol 2013; 130(3):652–659.
3. Smedley B, Jeffries M, Adelman L et al. Race, racial inequality and health inequities: separating myth from fact. Briefing paper, The Opportunity Agenda 2008. http://www.unnaturalcauses.org/assets/uploads/file/Race_Racial_Inequality_Health.pdf (Accessed August 17, 2017).
4. American Heart Association, African-Americans and Heart Disease, Stroke (2015). http://www.heart.org/HEARTORG/Conditions/More/MyHeartandStrokeNews/African-Americans-and-Heart-Disease_UCM_444863_Article.jsp#.WaMfSuNFySE (Accessed August 22, 2017).
5. Kumar B, Lenert P. Gout and African Americans: reducing disparities. Cleveland Clinic Journal of Medicine 2016; 83(9):665-674.
6. Silverberg JI. Racial and ethnic disparities in atopic dermatitis. Curr Dermatol Rep 2015; 4(1):44–48.
7. American College of Allergy. Asthma, and Immunology. Allergy Facts, 2015. Retrieved from: http://acaai.org/news/facts-statistics/allergies (Accessed April 19, 2018).
8. Fischer AH, Shin DB, Margolis DJ et al. Racial and ethnic differences in health care utilization for childhood eczema: An analysis of the 2001-2013 Medical Expenditure Panel Surveys. J Am Acad Dermatol 2017; 77(6):1060-1067. doi: 10.1016/j.jaad.2017.08.035.

9. United States Environmental Protection Agency, 2015. http://www.epa.gov/asthma/pdfs/asthma_fact_sheet_en.pdf (Accessed August 27, 2015).
10. Wegienka G, Havstad S, Joseph CL et al. Racial disparities in allergic outcomes in African Americans emerge as early as age 2 years. Clin Exp Allergy: Journal of the British Society for Allergy and Clinical Immunology. 2012; 42(6):909-917. doi:10.1111/j.1365-2222.2011.03946.x.
11. Cuatrescases P, Lockwood DH, Caldwell JR. Lactase deficiency in the adult. A common occurrence. Lancet 1965; 1(7375):14-8.
12. Maiyaki M, Garbati M. The burden of non-communicable diseases in Nigeria; in the context of globalization. Annals African Med 2014; 13(1), 1.
13. American Heart Association. High Blood Pressure and African Americans https://www.heart.org/en/health-topics/high-blood-pressure/why-high-blood-pressureis-a-silent-killer/high-blood-pressure-and-african-americans (Accessed August 3, 2019).
14. Beutler E, Duparc S. G6PD Deficiency Working Group. Glucose-6-phosphate dehydrogenase deficiency and antimalarial drug development. Am J Trop Med Hyg 2007; 77:779–89.
15. Centers for Disease Control and Prevention. Health, United States, 2015, With Special Feature on Racial and Ethnic Health Disparities (updated on June 22, 2017 to reflect corrections to the 2014 mortality data.) https://www.cdc.gov/nchs/data/hus/hus15.pdf
16. Centers for Disease Control and Prevention. Reproductive Health (Page last updated, September 28, 2016). https://www.cdc.gov/reproductivehealth/maternalinfanthealth/infantmortality.htm (Accessed, August 5, 2018).
17. Bryant AS, Worjoloh A, Caughey AB et al. Racial/ethnic disparities in obstetrical outcomes and care: prevalence and determinants. Am J Obstet Gynecol 2010; 202(4), 335–343.
18. March of Dimes, 2015. African-American. Fact Sheet (2015). https://www.marchofdimes.org/March-of-Dimes-Racial-and-Ethnic-Disparities_feb-27-2015.pdf (Accessed August 5, 2018).
19. CDC, 2018. Rates of maternal mortality are over twice those of women of European descent. https://www.cdc.gov/nchs/fastats/black-health.htm (Accessed August 19, 2019).
20. NCHS National Center for Health Statistics. Health, United States, 2015: With special feature on racial and ethnic health disparities. Hyattsville, MD: National Center for Health Statistics; 2016.

21. World Health Organization. Report on the status of major health risk factors for noncommunicable diseases: WHO 2016; ISBN 978-929023301-5.
https://afro.who.int/sites/default/files/2017-07/15264_who_afr-situation-ncds-15-12-2016-for-web.pdf (Accessed January 23, 2022).
22. Omar MAK, Seedat MA, Motala AA et al. The prevalence of diabetes mellitus and impaired glucose tolerance in a group of urban South African blacks. S Afr Med J 1993; 83:641-3.
23. Walker ARP, Sarell P. Coronary heart disease: outlook for Africa. J Roy Soc Med 1997; 90:23–27.
24. McCrae T. Osler's Principles and Practices of Medicine. London: Appleton, 1912:836.
25. Walker ARP. Cancer outlook: an African perspective. J Roy Soc Med 1995; 88:5-13.
26. Abrahams Z, Mchiza Z, Steyn NP. Diet and mortality rates in Sub-Saharan Africa: Stages in the nutrition transition. BMC Public Health 2011; 11:801. https://doi.org/10.1186/1471-2458-11-801

Notes

Further notes on health disparities: compared to European Americans, African Americans

- Are at higher risk for heart diseases, stroke, cancer, asthma, influenza and pneumonia, diabetes, and HIV/AIDS (1).
- Are more likely to die at younger ages from all causes (2), including diabetes and stroke (3).
- Have a three times higher rate of kidney failure (4) and account for a third of all patients in the U.S. receiving dialysis for kidney failure, but make up 12.7% of the U.S. population.
- Have the highest death rate and shortest survival from all cancers (5).
- Experienced more serious illness and death from COVID-19 during the 2021-2022 pandemic (6).

Additional References

1. Office of Minority Health Resource Center. "Profile: Black/African Americans." Black/African American - The Office of Minority Health, 22 Aug. 2019,
www.minorityhealth.hhs.gov/omh/browse.aspx?lvl=3&lvlid=61
2. "African American Health." Centers for Disease Control and Prevention, Centers for Disease Control and Prevention, 2 May 2017,

www.cdc.gov/vitalsigns/aahealth/infographic.html
3. "African-American Health Disparities." Cigna, Apr. 2016, www.cigna.com/health-care-providers/resources/african-american-black-health-disparities.
4. "African Americans and Kidney Disease." National Kidney Foundation, 16 Feb. 2018, www.kidney.org/news/newsroom/factsheets/African-Americans-and-CKD
5. American Cancer Society. Cancer Facts & Figures for African Americans 2019-2021.
6. "Coronavirus in African Americans and Other People of Color." Coronavirus in African Americans and Other People of Color | Johns Hopkins Medicine, Johns Hopkins Medicine, 20 Apr. 2020, www.hopkinsmedicine.org/health/conditions-and-diseases/coronavirus/covid19-racial-disparities.
https://www.pfizer.com/news/articles/health_disparities_among_african_americans

CHAPTER THREE

STRUCTURAL RACISM AND DISCRIMINATION

Health disparities are differences in disease incidence, prevalence, mortality, morbidity (complications), survivorship, including quality of life after treatment, burden of disease, and stage of disease at diagnosis.[1] Disparities in health and health care affecting African Americans are generally attributed to structural racism, which has created limited access to healthcare, poorer quality of healthcare, education, and housing, as well as stressful experiences related to racial discrimination, and poorer overall incomes. The continuing existence of discrimination, stress, and poorer healthcare is well documented.[2-4]

According to Williams et al.,[5] socioeconomic factors alone do not account for racial and ethnic inequities in health. Racism itself is a fundamental cause of adverse health outcomes for racial and ethnic minorities. For each of the primary domains of racism affecting mental and physical health outcomes – structural racism, cultural racism, and individual-level discrimination – Williams et al. present data and suggest priorities for future research to advance knowledge in the area.

The legacy of 400 years of slavery, violent oppression, discrimination, and emotional stress suffered by African Americans and the struggle both to receive and to provide health care, continues to have pervasive effects.[6-8] The COVID-19 pandemic in 2020-2022 has also disproportionately affected African Americans. Across the United States, COVID-19 mortality rates in predominantly black counties have been sixfold higher than in predominantly white counties.[9]

African Americans are also at increased risk of diabetes and its complications after controlling statistically for socioeconomic status.[10] Non-Hispanic black women have rates of preterm birth that are 40% higher than those of Hispanic and non-Hispanic white women after adjustment for maternal socioeconomic status and education.[11] Chronic worry about experiencing racial discrimination is reported to affect risks of premature birth among African American women, possibly through neuroendocrine, vascular or immune mechanisms involved in responses both to stress and the initiation of labor.[12] Such worry has been suggested to explain the puzzling observation of greater disparities in preterm birth among more socioeconomically-advantaged women.[13]

While disparities in access to and the quality of health care affecting African Americans remain rooted in structural racism and discrimination, the overall health profile of people of West Central African descent – showing both increased and reduced rates of death from different diseases – suggests a role for additional factors. For instance, in a 25-year follow-up study on the health of medical graduates, Black compared to White physicians had a higher risk of cardiovascular disease, with an earlier onset, twofold higher rates of diabetes and hypertension, a 40% higher rate of coronary artery disease, and a much higher case fatality rate of 52% vs. 9%.[14] Similarly, in a diverse cohort of 927 youth with type 1 diabetes, African Americans compared to other groups had a higher glycated hemoglobin (HbA1c) level after adjustment for many factors, higher rates of severe hypoglycemia and ketoacidosis, higher required doses of insulin per body weight, and a higher rate of hypertension. African American participants also had less residual β-cell function, which likely contributed to a worsened prognosis for type 1 diabetes.[15] Higher HbA1c levels are also reported in African American children with type 1 diabetes compared to white children, after adjustment for socioeconomic status, diabetes duration, and insulin dose.[16,17] After being diagnosed with type 1 diabetes, African American youth have unexplained adverse outcomes of earlier onset and prognosis for long-term complications.

A study of hypertension among West Africans in Africa and their descendants reported a stepwise increase in hypertension as groups moved from rural to urban Africa to the Caribbean, and from the Caribbean to the US. People of African descent in the US had hypertension levels that were twice as high as those in Africa, and higher than among mainly white populations in Europe.[18]

Another study comparing hypertension rates in West Africa, the Caribbean and the US, based on 10,014 individuals in seven locations and using standardized data collection methods, reported a consistent gradient of hypertension prevalence, rising from 16% in West Africa to 26% in the Caribbean and to 33% in the US. Mean blood pressures were similar among those aged 25 to 34 but the increase in rates of hypertension with age was twice as steep in the US as in Africa.[19]

Age-specific mortality rates from chronic diseases were often several-fold higher in younger black adult age-groups overall than in most high-income countries. Even more surprising, age-specific mortality rates from chronic diseases are higher in sub-Saharan Africa than in virtually all other regions of the world, both in men and women.[20]

These findings pose the following questions: How does the North American environment contribute to increased rates of chronic disease in all population groups that have been studied? Why are African Americans more susceptible to these diseases than European Americans? And why are chronic disease rates rising rapidly in Africa when they have historically been low? In short, why were Africans healthy in their original environment but unhealthier than Europeans in North America, and increasingly in Africa itself? In what way were Africans well-adapted health-wise in the West Central African environment, but fare less well in the United States? The thesis presented here suggests answers to these questions.

References

1. National Cancer Institute. Cancer Health Disparities. https://www.cancer.gov/aboutnci/organization/crchd/cancer-health-disparities-fact-sheet (Retrieved August 16, 2017).
2. Institute of Medicine. Unequal Treatment: confronting racial and ethnic disparities in health care. Washington, DC: National Academies Press, 2002.
3. LaVeist TA, Isaac LA (eds.) Race, Ethnicity and Health: A Public Health Reader, Second Edition. Jossey-Bass, San Francisco, 2013.
4. Assari S, Moazen-Zadeh E, Caldwell CH et al. Racial discrimination during adolescence predicts mental health deterioration in adulthood: gender differences among blacks. Front Public Health 2017; 5:104. doi: 10.3389/fpubh.2017.00104. eCollection 2017.
5. Williams DR, Lawrence JA, Davis BA. Racism and health: evidence and needed research. Ann Rev Public Health 2019; 40(1):105-125.
6. Braveman P, Gottlieb L. The social determinants of health: It's time to consider the causes of the causes. Public Health Rep 2014;129(2):19–31.
7. Colen CG, Ramey DM, Cooksey EC et al. Racial disparities in health among nonpoor African Americans and Hispanics: The role of acute and chronic discrimination. Soc Sci Med 2017. pii: S0277-9536(17)30290-3. doi: 10.1016/j.socscimed.2017.04.051.
8. deShazo RD (ed). The Racial Divide in American Medicine: Black Physicians and the Struggle for Justice in Health Care. University Press of Mississippi, Jackson, 2018.
9. Yancy CW. COVID-19 and African Americans. JAMA 2020; 323:1891–1892.

10. Williams DR, Priest N, Anderson NB. Understanding associations among race, socioeconomic status, and health: Patterns and prospects. Health Psychol 2016;35(4):407–411. doi:10.1037/hea0000242.
11. Behrman RE, Butler AS, Eds., in Preterm Birth: Causes, Consequences, and Prevention.The National Academies Press, Washington, DC, 2006.
12. Dominguez TP. Adverse birth outcomes in African American women: The social context of persistent reproductive disadvantage. Social Work in Public Health 2011: 26(1):3-16.
DOI: 10.1080/10911350902986880
13. Braveman P, Heck K, Egerter S et al. Worry about racial discrimination: A missing piece of the puzzle of Black-White disparities in preterm birth? PLoS One 2017;12(10):e0186151. doi:
10.1371/journal.pone.0186151. eCollection 2017.
14. Thomas J, Thomas DJ, Pearson T et al. Cardiovascular disease in African American and white physicians: the Meharry Cohort and Meharry-Hopkins Cohort Studies. J Health Care Poor Underserved. 1997 Aug;8(3):270-83; discussion 284. doi: 10.1353/hpu.2010.0526. PMID: 9253218.
15. Redondo MJ, Libman I, Cheng P et al. Racial/ethnic minority youth with recent-onset Type 1 diabetes have poor prognostic factors. Diabetes Care 2018; 41(5):1017-1024; DOI: 10.2337/dc17-2335
16. Delamater AM, Albrecht DR, Postellon DC et al. Racial differences in metabolic control of children and adolescents with type I diabetes mellitus. Diabetes Care 1991;14:20–25.
17. Bell RA, Mayer-Davis EJ, Beyer JW, et al.; SEARCH for Diabetes in Youth Study Group. Diabetes in non-Hispanic white youth: prevalence, incidence, and clinical characteristics: the SEARCH for Diabetes in Youth study. Diabetes Care 2009;32(Suppl. 2):S102–S111.
18. Cooper R, Rotimi C, Ataman S et al. The prevalence of hypertension in seven populations of west African origin. Am J Public Health 1997; 87(2):160–168.
18A. Cooper R, Rotimi C. Hypertension in blacks. Am J Hypertens 1997; 10(7 Pt 1):804-12.
20. de-Graft Aikins A, Unwin N et al., Agyemang C, Allotey P, Campbell C, Arhinful D. Tackling Africa's chronic disease burden: from the local to the global. Globalization and Health 2010; 6(1). DOI: 10.1186/1744-8603-6-5

Notes

A summary of "Systemic Racism and Health Disparities: A Statement from the Editors of Family Medicine Journals". Sumi M. Sexton, MD, American Family Physician and other editors. Published ahead of print, October 15, 2020: https://www.aafp.org/pubs/afp/content/Racism_statement.html

The year 2020 was marked by historic protests following the deaths of George Floyd, Ahmaud Arbery, Breonna Taylor, and many other Black people. These protests heightened awareness of racism as a public health crisis, its profound adverse effects on physical and mental health, (1,2) and on negative patient experiences in the healthcare system.(3,4) They noted that race is a sociopolitical construct that continues to disadvantage Black and other People of Color, (5-8) and to affirm that family medicine is a specialty that has emerged as a counterculture to reform mainstream medicine, (9) – both to confront systemic racism and eliminate health disparities – "so we can better serve our patients and our communities."

Additional References

1. Institute of Medicine (US) Committee on Understanding and Eliminating Racial and Ethnic Disparities in Health Care, Smedley BD, Stith AY, Nelson AR, eds. Unequal treatment: confronting racial and ethnic disparities in health care. Washington, DC: National Academies Press; 2003.
2. Bailey ZD, Krieger N, Agénor M, Graves J, Linos N, Bassett MT. Structural racism and health inequities in the USA: evidence and interventions. Lancet. 2017;389(10077):1453-1463.
3. Ben J, Cormack D, Harris R, Paradies Y. Racism and health service utilisation: A systematic review and meta-analysis. PLoS One. 2017;12(12):e0189900.
4. Paradies Y, Ben J, Denson N, et al. Racism as a determinant of health: a systematic review and meta-analysis. PLoS One. 2015;10(9):e0138511.
5. American Academy of Family Physicians. Institutional racism in the health care system. Published 2019. Accessed Sept. 15, 2020. https://www.aafp.org/about/policies/all/institutional-racism.html
6. Yaya S, Yeboah H, Charles CH, Otu A, Labonte R. Ethnic and racial disparities in COVID-19-related deaths: counting the trees, hiding the forest. BMJ Glob Health. 2020;5(6):e002913.

7. Egede LE, Walker RJ. Structural Racism, Social Risk Factors, and Covid-19 — A Dangerous Convergence for Black Americans [published online ahead of print, 2020 Jul 22]. N Engl J Med. 2020;10.1056/NEJMp2023616.
8. Centers for Disease Control and Prevention. Health equity considerations and racial and ethnic minority groups. Updated July 24, 2020. Accessed Sept. 15, 2020. https://www.cdc.gov/coronavirus/2019-ncov/community/health-equity/race-ethnicity.html
9. Stephens GG. Family medicine as counterculture. Fam Med. 1989;21(2):103-109.

Professor Paula Lantz, University of Michigan, writes that growing numbers of states have banned the teaching of Critical Race Theory (CRT) and other frameworks about structural racism in K-12 schools. Her view is that the scientific tenets that underlie CRT are crucial for understanding and addressing racial inequality in important social outcomes, including population health; and CRT provides a framework for understanding racial inequality, supported by decades of multidisciplinary scholarship. The tenets of CRT are essential in seeking to address racial inequalities in all social outcomes, and that "there can be no objective or effective teaching, research, or practice addressing the large racial health disparities (e.g., in life expectancy, infant/maternal mortality, and almost every type of illness or injury) that persist in the U.S. that does not implicitly or explicitly incorporate the main tenets of CRT."

Regarding population health science, these tenets are: 1) Race is a social construction in the way that race is defined and experienced and is the result of social and political thought and actions that change over time. "Race" is not a biological imperative driving disease processes and longevity, but rather a marker for how individuals experience physical and social exposures, including discrimination, that influence health over the life course. 2) Racism and its outcomes are perpetuated through social processes above and beyond individual actions through cultural norms, institutional rules, and laws and regulations. Racism as not primarily person to person, but rather the processes built into institutions, systems, and policies that reinforce, codify, and perpetuate exposures and opportunities that differ across socioeconomic and racial groups. 3) Because racism is commonplace, understanding structural racism within our institutions and policies – on education, income, housing, food, criminal justice, the environment, and health care – are key for addressing population health inequities. 4) Listening to and understanding the lived experiences of individuals is essential for understanding how racism works to create inequities in individual outcomes, including health, and that there is a need to better represent in research, the media, and policy reform work, how racism in all its manifestations is experienced by people in ways that matter, including for physical/mental health. Lantz concludes that those committed to health equity through population health science should publicly defend the tenets of CRT and their long-standing contributions to population health in teaching, research, community-based efforts and policy reform, to improve health and well-being for all. (Professor Lantz defends Critical Race Theory, May 2022 https://fordschool.umich.edu/news/2022/lantz-defends-critical-race-theory)

CHAPTER FOUR

OTHER CLUES TO EXPLAINING HEALTH DISPARITIES

Health Disparities in the Reverse Direction

A major clue in explaining the origin and causes of health disparities affecting African Americans is that disparities also exist in the reverse direction; that is, people of West Central African descent are protected from severe disease and less likely than European Americans to die from malaria, yellow fever, and dengue hemorrhagic fever.[1-4] In earlier centuries, African workers were highly prized in the Caribbean because they were less likely than Europeans to succumb to these diseases, all of which were highly prevalent and lethal in the region at the time.[5] African Americans are also at lower risk of non-alcoholic fatty liver disease (NAFLD),[6,7] which is defined as hepatic fat accumulation (steatosis) >5% of total weight of the liver and affects >30% or more of older European Americans.[8] African Americans have less hepatic lipid content, lower plasma lipoprotein lipase, and less overall liver disease.[9] NAFLD is a growing global epidemic, affecting millions of people worldwide. The burden of NAFLD is widely underestimated.[10] In the US, Hispanics are the most disproportionately affected whereas African Americans as a group are least affected by hepatic steatosis and elevated aminotransferase enzyme levels. Considering the vital role of the liver in metabolism and in overall health, the anomaly of lower rates of NAFLD in African Americans suggests an underlying biological process or mechanism related to the liver, which potentially explains the pattern of health disparities affecting African Americans.

African Americans also have the lowest risk of osteoporosis of any racial group at younger ages, as well as higher bone densities and lower bone turnover rates,[11 (p. 71)] and have half the nonvertebral fracture rate of European Americans.[12,13] However, when hip fractures do occur, African American women are more likely to die than European American women; they also have longer hospital stays and are less likely to be ambulatory at discharge.[14]

The thesis proposed here is that differences in health outcomes affecting African Americans, both negative and positive, are due in part to evolutionary physiological adaptations to the ancestral environment of West Central Africa. This environment was and remains broadly characterized by exposure to potentially lethal parasitic (protozoan and helminthic) organisms, most notably those causing malaria, schistosomiasis, and onchocerciasis.[15] It is suggested that these adaptations were successful in enhancing survival in the original ancestral environment, but they are potentially disadvantageous in the environment of North America, as explained below.

About 3.3 billion people are at risk of malaria due to *Plasmodium falciparum*, the most dangerous malaria parasite, making it one of the world's most significant health problems.[16] There were 214 million new cases of malaria worldwide in 2015, with Africa accounting for most (88%), and an estimated 438,000 deaths from malaria worldwide, mostly in Africa (90%) and in children under age 6, i.e., about 0.2% of the 214 million cases, indicating the comparative rarity of lethal outcomes.[17]

Schistosoma mansoni, a waterborne flatworm trematode parasite known as a schistosome, is the leading cause of schistosomiasis and the second most common human parasitic disease after malaria. It is found in areas with water contaminated with freshwater snails, the intermediate host for the parasites. The disease causes liver and intestinal damage and the worms can live in the bloodstream for decades, even if the host has a healthy immune system. In 2016, 207 million people in 75 countries had the disease and about 200,000 people, mostly in Africa, died from it.[18]

Onchocerca volvulus, also known as "river blindness", is a filarial (arthropod-borne) nematode (roundworm) that causes onchocerciasis, the second leading infectious cause of blindness worldwide after trachoma. The disease is transmitted by repeated bites from blackflies that live near fast-flowing streams and rivers in remote rural areas. In addition to causing visual impairment that can progress to blindness, onchocerciasis is also associated with severe skin disease, including intense itching, skin atrophy, rashes, or nodules under the skin. About 18 million people are affected by the disease.[19]

Environmental Exposure to Vitamin A-Ingesting Pathogens

A second major clue to explaining the health profile of people of West Central Africa is that both *P. falciparum*[20] and *Onchocerciasis volvulus*[21] selectively absorb vitamin A from the human host. Mizuno et al.

investigated the uptake of vitamin A by culturing a standard isolate of the parasite (FCR-3) with 3H-labelled vitamin A, at concentrations of the vitamin corresponding to those normally present in human serum. They found that the 3H-labelled vitamin A accumulated in the parasites from each culture in a parasitemia-dependent manner and that the radioactivity detected in the parasites increased with parasite maturation from the ring to the late-trophozoite stage.[20] In the case of *Onchocercus volvulus*, a study of infected patients showed that while the median tissue retinol concentration was 1.4 IU/ml (range: 0.8-1.9), that of four batches of adult whole worms, derived from four different individuals, was 12.6 IU/g (range: 1.6-39.7) – eight times higher on average that in the skin.[21]

Vitamin A is a major potential toxin and there is evidence that its use in parasite reproduction causes the signs and symptoms of the respective diseases. (For further details on vitamin A in malaria and onchocerciasis, see Other Essays).

In the case of trematode parasites, including *Schistosoma japonicum*, the major active vitamin A metabolite retinoic acid (RA) is actively taken up by the parasitic nematode *Brugia Malaya*,[22] and vitamin A signaling pathways are involved.[23] It is not known if schistosoma selectively absorb vitamin A. However, significant reductions in serum vitamin A, zinc and carotenoids were observed in patients with active *Schistosoma mansoni* infection and complications of the disease, including anemia,[24] suggesting that the parasite selectively absorbs vitamin A from the host.

It is proposed that use of the ingested vitamin A in parasite reproduction also contributes to the signs and symptoms of the respective diseases – malaria, schistosomiasis, and onchocerciasis – all of which represent endogenous forms of hypervitaminosis A (i.e., vitamin A poisoning).[25-27] Over the course of millennia, the people of West Central Africa adapted physiologically to the toxic effects of vitamin A, resulting from its uptake and use by the parasites. Here the pathogenesis of malaria is first outlined, followed by a summary of the biochemistry of vitamin A (Chapter 5).

The Pathogenesis of Malaria

Malaria parasites spend more than a week in the host liver before emerging in the form of merozoites and invading the red blood cells (RBCs).[28] I have hypothesized that the merozoite-stage parasites, on leaving the liver packed with vitamin A, use it as a cell membrane destabilizer to invade and reproduce in the RBCs.[27] As the damaged RBCs begin to die, their contents of vitamin A are released into the circulation, causing the signs and symptoms of the disease as endogenous form of hypervitaminosis

A. The features of malaria include fever, flu-like illness, fatigue, headache, muscle aches, gastrointestinal symptoms, respiratory distress, anemia, jaundice, and retinopathy, progressing to seizures and coma with worsening severity. These features closely resemble those of vitamin A toxicity.

In patients with malaria who are pregnant, vitamin A compounds released from damaged RBCs enter the fetus and are hypothesized to cause preterm birth and/or fetal growth restriction as a function of the membrane-destabilizing and growth-inhibiting effects of vitamin A. Obesity, both alone and in combination with additional metabolic risk factors (hypertension, dyslipidemia, or diabetes), is strongly associated with severe malaria[29] and may increase susceptibility to the disease due to greater accumulation of vitamin A in the liver.

The proposed vitamin A toxicity hypothesis of the pathogenesis of malaria has been supported by the results of a Korean study comparing vitamin A profiles in patients infected with *Plasmodium vivax* (PV, n = 74) with those of non-malarial patients with fever (n=25). As predicted, the PV patients had significantly lower serum levels of retinol but higher levels of retinoic acid.[30]

Most discussions of malaria include the signs and symptoms of the disease but the actual mechanism of death from malaria has remained uncertain. I have proposed that death is not due directly to the parasites themselves but to their use of the vitamin A, absorbed from the human host, in the course of reproduction; that is, its release into the circulation from dying red blood cells in toxic concentrations. This model, now supported by the results of the Korean study, has implications for prevention and treatment but they remain to be recognized and implemented.

In summary, the proposed model is that the features of malaria represent an endogenous form of vitamin A poisoning, arising from use of the host's own stores of vitamin A by *P. falciparum* to complete its life cycle. Hence, reduced background liver reserves of vitamin A would be expected to reduce the severity of malaria. This situation appears to apply to populations exposed to malaria parasitism in West Central Africa. Conversely, high background levels, e.g., associated with fatty liver disease, would be expected to increase disease severity and lethality, related to its increased availability for use by the parasites following infection. This situation appears to apply to people of European descent.

References

1. Adu B, Dodoo D, Adukpo S, Gyan BA, Hedley PL, Goka B, et al. (2011) Polymorphisms in the RNASE3 Gene Are Associated with

Susceptibility to Cerebral Malaria in Ghanaian Children. PLoS ONE 6(12): e29465. https://doi.org/10.1371/journal.pone.0029465
2. Gainor EM, Harris E, LaBeaud AD. Uncovering the Burden of Dengue in Africa: Considerations on Magnitude, Misdiagnosis, and Ancestry. Viruses. 2022 Jan 25;14(2):233. doi: 10.3390/v14020233. PMID: 35215827; PMCID: PMC8877195.
3. Sierra B, Kouri G, Guzman MG. Race: a risk factor for dengue hemorrhagic fever. Arch Virol 2007; 52:533-543.
4. McGuire RA, Coelho PRP. Parasites, Pathogens, and Progress: Diseases and Economic Development. Cambridge, MA: MIT Press, 2011. DOI: https://doi.org/10.7551/mitpress/9780262015660.001.0001
5. Blake LE, Garcia-Blancoa MA. Human genetic variation and yellow fever mortality during 19th century U.S. epidemics. mBio 2014; 5(3). e01253-14 https://doi.org/10.1128/mBio.01253-14
6. Samji NS, Snell PD, Singal AK et al. Racial Disparities in Diagnosis and Prognosis of Nonalcoholic Fatty Liver Disease. Clinical Liver Disease 2020; 16:66-72. https://doi.org/10.1002/cld.948
7. Guerrero R, Vega GL, Grundy SM et al. Ethnic differences in hepatic steatosis: An insulin resistance paradox? Hepatology 2009; 49:791–801. doi:10.1002/hep.22726.
8. Dongiovanni P, Anstee Q, Valenti L. Genetic predisposition in NAFLD and NASH: Impact on severity of liver disease and response to treatment. Curr Pharm Design 2013; 19(29), 5219–5238.
9. Sumner AE, Harman JL, Buxbaum SG et al. The triglyceride/high-density lipoprotein cholesterol ratio fails to predict insulin resistance in African-American women: an analysis of Jackson Heart Study. Metab Syndr Relat Disord 2010; 8(6):511-4.
10. Sherif ZA, Saeed A, Ghavimi S, et al. Global epidemiology of nonalcoholic fatty liver disease and perspectives on US minority populations. Dig Dis Sci 2016; 61(5):1214-25. doi: 10.1007/s10620-016-4143-0.
11. Overfield T. Biological variation in health and illness: Race, age and sex differences. 2nd Edition. CRC Press, Boca Raton, FL. 1995.
12. Weinstein RS, Bell NH. Diminished rates of bone formation in normal black adults. N Engl J Med 1988; 319(26):1698-701.
13. Griffin MR, Ray WA, Fought RL et al. Black-white differences in fracture rates. Am J Epidemiol 1992; 136(11): 1378-85.
14. Cauley JA. Defining ethnic and racial differences in osteoporosis and fragility fractures. Clin Orthop Rel Res 2011; 469(7):1891-1899. doi:10.1007/s11999-011-1863-5.

15. Cummings R, Turco S. Parasitic Infections. In: Varki A, Cummings RD, Esko JD, et al., editors. Essentials of Glycobiology. 2nd edition. Cold Spring Harbor (NY): Cold Spring Harbor Laboratory Press, 2009, Chapter 40. Available from: https://www.ncbi.nlm.nih.gov/books/NBK1899/
16. Crawley J, Chu C, Mtove G et al. Malaria in children. Lancet 2010; 375:1468-1481.
17. WHO 2018. World Malaria Report. https://apps.who.int/iris/bitstream/handle/10665/275867/9789241565653-eng.pdf?ua=1 (Accessed November 1, 2020).
18. Global Burden of Disease. Disease and Injury Incidence and Prevalence, Collaborators. Global, regional, and national incidence, prevalence, and years lived with disability for 310 diseases and injuries, 1990-2015: a systematic analysis for the Global Burden of Disease Study 2015. Lancet 2016; 388 (10053):1545–1602. doi:10.1016/S0140-6736(16)31678-6.
19. CDC, 2018. Parasites – Onchocerciasis (also known as River Blindness) https://www.cdc.gov/parasites/onchocerciasis/index.html (Accessed November 1, 2020).
20. Mizuno Y, Kawazu SI, Kano S et al. In-vitro uptake of vitamin A by Plasmodium falciparum. Annals Trop Med Parasitol 2003; 97:237–43.
21. Stürchler D, Wyss F, Hanck A. Retinol, onchocerciasis and Onchocerca volvulus. Trans R Soc Trop Med Hyg 1981;75(4):617–617.
22. Wolff KM, Scott AL. Brugia malayi: retinoic acid uptake and localization. Exp Parasitol 1995; 80:282–90.
23. Qiu C, Fu Z, Shi Y et al. A retinoid X receptor (RXR1) homolog from Schistosoma japonicum: its ligand-binding domain may bind to 9-cis-retinoic acid. Mol Biochem Parasitol 2013; 188(1):40-50. doi: 10.1016/j.molbiopara.2013.02.002.
24. Mikhail MM, Mansour MM. Complications of human schistosomiasis and their effect on levels of plasma copper, zinc and serum vitamin A. Hum Nutr Clin Nutr 1982; 36(4):289-96.
25. Mawson AR, WaKabongo M. Onchocerciasis-associated morbidity: hypothesis. Trans Roy Soc Trop Med Hyg 2002; 96:1-2.
26. Mawson AR, Makunde WH, Penman AD et al. Retinoid expression in onchocercal skin disease: pilot study. Infect Dis (Auckl) 2017; 10:1178633617731741. doi: 10.1177/1178633617731741. eCollection 2017.
27. Mawson AR. The pathogenesis of malaria: a new perspective. Pathogens Global Health 2013; 107(3), 122–129.
28. Milner DA Jr. Malaria Pathogenesis. Cold Spring Harb Perspect Med. 2018 Jan 2;8(1):a025569. doi: 10.1101/cshperspect.a025569.

29. Wyss K, Wångdahl A, Vesterlund M, et al. Obesity and diabetes as risk factors for severe Plasmodium falciparum malaria: results from a Swedish nationwide study. Clin Infect Dis 2017; 65(6):949-958. doi:10.1093/cid/cix437.
30. Na J, Khan A, Kim JK, Wadood A, Choe YL, Walker DI, Jones DP, Lim CS, Park YH. Discovery of metabolic alterations in the serum of patients infected with Plasmodium spp. by high-resolution metabolomics. Metabolomics. 2019 Dec 23;16(1):9. doi: 10.1007/s11306-019-1630-2. PMID: 31872321.

Notes

Please see Other Essays, 1 and 2.

CHAPTER FIVE

VITAMIN A (RETINOIDS)

Retinoids are natural and synthetic forms of vitamin A; that is, compounds derived from vitamin A or similar to it in structure. Vitamin A is derived from the diet either "preformed", from vegetables and fruits, as beta-carotene and other carotenoids, and then converted to vitamin A in the body, or as "provitamin A", which derives directly from animal sources. Carotene-rich plants include dark-green leafy vegetables, deep yellow, red, green and orange peppers and fruits, sweet potatoes, carrots, pumpkin and other winter squashes, cantaloupe, apricots, peaches, and mangoes. Dietary sources of preformed vitamin A as retinyl palmitate include beef, calf, and chicken liver, eggs, fish liver oils, and dairy products such as milk, whole milk yogurt and cottage cheese, other cheeses, and butter.[1]

Vitamin A is considered essential in very low concentration for numerous biological functions, including immunity, cellular growth, development, and reproduction.[2] However, in higher concentration retinoids are cytotoxic, mutagenic and teratogenic.[3,4]

Serum retinol level, the primary indicator of vitamin A nutritional status, it is controlled homeostatically by the liver and does not decline until body stores are almost depleted. It also declines in response to acute and chronic infections and is therefore unreliable, by itself, for determining the vitamin A status of individuals or the impact of interventions.[5,6] Combinations of retinol and retinyl esters and their ratios, along with retinoic acid, provide more precise measures of overall vitamin A status, including toxicity, but neither retinyl esters nor retinoic acid are measured routinely in clinical practice.

Retinoic acid (RA), the main active metabolite, is produced from retinol via hydrolysis of retinyl esters (REs) in the liver (see Figure 2).

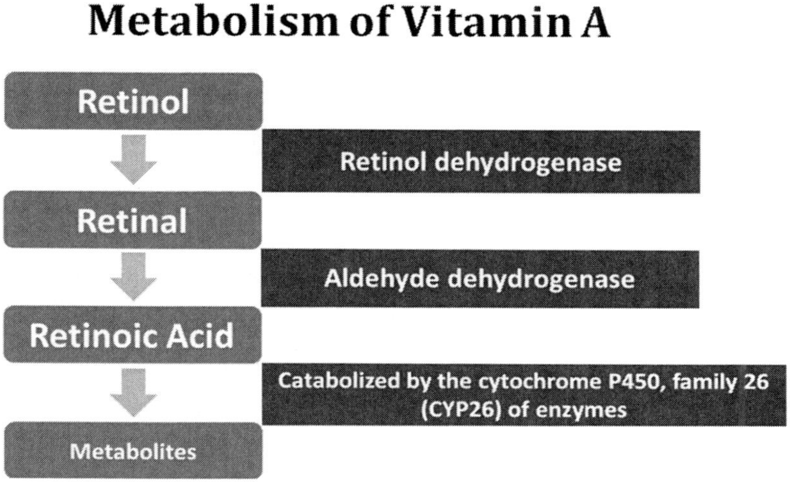

Figure 2. Metabolism of vitamin A

Retinol is delivered to the target tissues bound to protein, as retinol-binding protein4 (RBP4) and is oxidized to retinal (retinaldehyde) via alcohol dehydrogenase. RA is synthesized from retinaldehyde via an aldehyde dehydrogenase reaction and exerts its numerous effects by controlling the expression of over 500 genes through binding to and activating the nuclear protein receptors: retinoic acid receptors (RARs) and retinoid X receptors (RXRs).[7]

About 80% of vitamin A is stored in the liver in the form of retinyl esters, in quantities sufficient to last the average adult about two years without the need for additional intake.[8] Lesser quantities are stored in the lung, adipose tissue, and intestine. It can be toxic if released into the circulation unbound to protein, as retinyl esters (REs) or retinoic acid. Toxicity can result from excessive dietary intake, dietary supplements, food supplemented with vitamin A, and vitamin A medications; it can also occur when the liver becomes saturated with vitamin A and stored REs spill into the circulation.

Unbound REs destroy cell membranes and are a major source of vitamin A toxicity. RA is up to 100 times more biologically active and hence more toxic than retinol. An autopsy study aimed at evaluating serum REs as a biomarker of vitamin A status against total liver reserves (TLRs, the gold standard), suggested that 7.5% total serum vitamin A as retinyl esters (and 3 μmol/g liver) is diagnostic for toxicity at the individual level in adults. In this study, serum RE concentrations were strongly correlated with TLRs; nine subjects (33%) had hypervitaminosis A ($\geq$1.0 μmol vitamin A/g liver), two of whom had >7.5% total serum vitamin A as REs; liver histology corroborated toxicity at 3 μmol/g liver; and no subject had >10% total serum vitamin A as REs.[9] The authors concluded that while the long-term impact of vitamin A supplements and fortificants on vitamin A status is currently unknown, "Considering the high prevalence of hypervitaminotic TLRs in this cohort, and given that many countries are adding preformed vitamin A to processed products, population biomarkers diagnosing hypervitaminosis before toxicity are urgently needed."

Acute vitamin A toxicity is characterized by fever, nausea and vomiting, headache, fatigue, blurred vision, lack of muscular coordination and skin peeling, associated with mitochondrial dysfunction. Early symptoms of chronic vitamin A toxicity are alopecia, dry eyes, severe headache, and generalized weakness. Later changes include cortical hyperostosis of bone and arthralgia, fractures, pruritus, failure to thrive in infants, hepatomegaly and splenomegaly.[10-12] Intakes of vitamin A only marginally above the recommended amount in early pregnancy (7,800 μg/day) are associated with congenital malformations.[13]

In a study showing that chronic consumption of vitamin A can impair bone formation in children, Zambian children with a high prevalence of hypervitaminosis A were recruited into an intervention study that included vitamin A at the recommended level, as retinyl palmitate or a placebo, for 90 days. It was found that bone formation was strongly improved in the placebo group consuming low preformed vA.[14]

A variety of infections associated with transient increases in C-reactive protein (CRP) and α-1-acid glycoprotein (AGP) are also associated with declines in retinol-binding protein (RBP) and plasma retinol concentrations.[15,16] The latter findings have been interpreted as signs of deficiency, but overall vitamin A nutritional status remains unclear in response to inflammation; in particular, retinyl ester and retinoic acid concentrations have not been measured. However, in a study of experimentally-induced *Escherichia coli* mastitis in heifers, the infection was associated with increased fever and decreased serum retinol but with significant increases in all-trans-retinoic acid. These changes in vitamin A concentration profiles during infection argue against a deficiency state and instead suggest a profound shift in retinoid metabolism towards the active metabolite, retinoic acid;[17] that is, to a state of retinoid toxicity.

As noted by an expert on vitamin in a commentary decades ago: "People seem reluctant to recognize just how toxic is vitamin A. Considered as a chronic poison, vitamin A is probably more harmful than cyanide … Vitamin A is an essential substance … But it is a very dangerous substance and it needs to be handled with care."[18]

References

1. Vitamin A and Carotenoids. Fact Sheet for Health Professionals https://ods.od.nih.gov/factsheets/VitaminA-HealthProfessional/ (Accessed December 16, 2022).
2. Ross AC. Vitamin A. In: Ross AC, Caballero B, Cousins RJ, Tucker KL, Ziegler TR, eds. Modern Nutrition in Health and Disease. 11th ed. Baltimore, MD: Lippincott Williams & Wilkins; 2014:260-77.
3. D'Ambrosio DN, Clugston RD, Blaner WS. Vitamin A metabolism: an update. Nutrients 2011; 3(1):63-103. doi: 10.3390/nu3010063.
4. Li Y, Wongsiriroj N, Blaner WS. The multifaceted nature of retinoid transport and metabolism. Hepatobiliary Surg Nutr 2014; 3(3):126-139. doi: 10.3978/j.issn.2304-3881.2014.05.04
5. Stephenson CB. Vitamin A, infection, and immune function. Annu Rev Nutr 2001; 21:167-192. www.annualreviews.org
6. WHO. Serum retinol concentrations for determining the prevalence of vitamin A deficiency in populations. Vitamin and Mineral Nutrition Information System. Geneva, World Health Organization, 2011 (WHO/NMH/NHD/MNM/11.3) (http://www.who.int/vmnis/indicators/retinol.pdf Accessed November 1, 2020).
7. Theodosiou M, Laudet V, Schubert M. From carrot to clinic: an overview of the retinoic acid signaling pathway. Cell Mol Life Sci 2010: 67:1423–1445. www.oalib.com/references/9073639
8. De Luca LM, Creek KE. Vitamin A and the liver. Prog Liver Dis 1986; 8:81–98.
9. Olsen K, Suri DJ, Davis C et al. Serum retinyl esters are positively correlated with analyzed total liver vitamin A reserves collected from US adults at time of death. Am J Clin Nutr 2018; 108(5):997–1005. https://doi.org/10.1093/ajcn/nqy190
10. Penniston KL, Tanumihardjo SA. The acute and chronic toxic effects of vitamin A. Am J Clin Nutr 2006; 83:191–201.
11. de Oliveira MR, Da Rocha RF, Pasquali MA, Moreira JC. The effects of vitamin A supplementation for 3 months on adult rat nigrostriatal axis: increased monoamine oxidase enzyme activity, mitochondrial redox dysfunction, increased β-amyloid(1–40) peptide and TNF-α contents, and susceptibility of mitochondria to an in vitro H2O2 challenge. Brain Res Bull 2012; 87:432–44.
12. de Oliveira MR. Vitamin A and retinoids as mitochondrial toxicants. Oxid Med Cell Longev 2015; 2015:140267. doi: 10.1155/2015/140267.

13. Allen L, Haskell M. Estimating the potential for vitamin A toxicity in women and young children. J Nutr 2002; 132:2907S-2919S.
14. Tanumihardjo SA, Gannon BM, Kaliwile C et al. Restricting vitamin A intake increases bone formation in Zambian children with high liver stores of vitamin. Arch Osteoporos 2019; 14(1):72. doi: 10.1007/s11657-019-0617-y. PMID: 31254130; PMCID:PMC7189610.
15. Thurnham DI, McCabe GP, Northrop-Clewes CA, Nestel P. Effects of subclinical infection on plasma retinol concentrations and assessment of prevalence of vitamin A deficiency: meta-analysis. Lancet 2003; 362(9401):2052-8. doi: 10.1016/s0140-6736(03)15099-4.
16. Larson LM, Namaste SM, Williams AM, Engle-Stone R, Addo OY, Suchdev PS, Wirth JP, Temple V, Serdula M, Northrop-Clewes CA. Adjusting retinol-binding protein concentrations for inflammation: Biomarkers Reflecting Inflammation and Nutritional Determinants of Anemia (BRINDA) project. Am J Clin Nutr 2017 Jul; 106(Suppl 1):390S-401S. doi: 10.3945/ajcn.116.142166.
17. Merris E van, Meyer E, Duchateau L et al. All-trans-retinoic acid is increased in the acute phase-related hyporetinemia during Escherichia coli mastitis. J Dairy Sci 2004; 87:980-987.
18. Pitt GAJ. Vitamin efficiency and excess. In Taylor TG, ed. The importance of vitamins to human Health. Baltimore, MD: University Park Press, 1979, pp. 81-90.

CHAPTER SIX

ADAPTATIONS TO VITAMIN A-INGESTING ORGANISMS

Evidence was presented in Chapter 4 that the malaria parasite, the onchocerciasis-causing helminthic nematode, and schistosome flatworms all absorb vitamin A from the host, and its use in reproduction contributes to the respective diseases. In what way, then, are people of West Central African descent protected from malaria in being less likely to die from the disease than people of European descent?

It is proposed that over the course of millennia, West Central Africans adapted physiologically to the threat of lethal parasitic infection in at least two ways:

1) Vitamin A was gradually sequestered away from the liver to other tissues to reduce its accessibility to the parasite and thereby prevent its use in reproduction and in causing disease.
2) The enzymatic metabolism of vitamin A was slowed, causing it to accumulate to sub-toxic levels and weaken the parasite, thereby reducing the potential lethality of the disease.

Sequestering Vitamin A Away from the Liver to Other Tissues

Little is known at present about the distribution of vitamin A in different tissues, particularly in relation to ancestral origin. With regard to abdominal adipose tissue, European Americans have an increased *s* (VAT) mass, which is strongly related to liver fat[1] and to hepatic vitamin A accumulation,[2] compared to African Americans, whereas the latter have greater *subcutaneous* abdominal adipose tissue (SAT) mass compared to European Americans.[3] Adipose tissue is an important storage site for retinol, containing an estimated 10–20% of total vitamin A in the body as retinyl esters.[4] The importance of vitamin A in adipose tissue and its role in the development of obesity and type 2 diabetes has become increasingly apparent.[5] Both aldehyde dehydrogenase and retinaldehyde dehydrogenase are responsible for catalyzing the first and second steps in the oxidation of retinol to retinal and retinoic acid, respectively, and have been identified in adipose tissue.[6]

African Americans have the highest mortality and the lowest survival of any racial/ethnic group for most cancers. During the most recent 5-year period, African American men had a 6% higher incidence rate but a 19% higher mortality than European American men overall, and an approximately 2-fold higher risk of death from myeloma, stomach cancer, and prostate cancer. African American women have an 8% lower overall incidence rate than White women overall, but a 12% higher mortality rate, including a two-fold higher mortality rate for endometrial cancer and a 41% higher rate for breast cancer, despite similar or lower incidence rates. Breast cancer surpassed lung cancer as the leading cause of cancer death among Black women in 2019.[7]

The proposed theory is that people of sub-Saharan African descent have higher concentrations of vitamin A in tissues outside the liver than people of European descent, and in the tissues to which African Americans are at increased risk of various diseases compared to European Americans.

Lung cancer is the leading cause of cancer deaths, disproportionately affecting African Americans.[8] Stellate (vitamin A-containing) storage cells are present not only in subcutaneous abdominal tissue but also in kidneys and lung.[9] However, the lung content and possible role of vitamin A in the disparity in lung cancer appears to be unknown. The same applies to other tissue diseases and disparities affecting African Americans. Although vitamin A deficiency in the lung is a focus of current research,[10] accumulating evidence indicates that a diet high in fat (and by implication, vitamin A) content is closely associated with prostate cancer progression in particular.[11,12] A study of prostate cancer in relation to diet among US citizens and Canadians of African, European, and Asian descent showed that fat intake and percentage of energy from fat differed among different ethnicities and were highest in those of African descent followed by those of European, Japanese, and Chinese ancestry.[13] A one-to-one, age- and race-matched case-control study involving 181 histologically confirmed cases of prostate cancer in African American patients and 181 controls showed that risk enhancement was associated with increased intake of proteins, total fat, saturated fat, oleic acid, and vitamin A. The association was highly significant for vitamin A, and a hypothesis based on disturbance of the zinc-retinol binding protein-vitamin A axis was proposed to explain the relative risk enhancement effect of vitamin A on prostate cancer.[14]

Dietary intake also plays a role in the rarity of colon cancer in black Africans (prevalence < 1:100,000) compared to white South Africans (17 per 100,000 population). Measures of food consumption and cancer risk in

Black and White adult South Africans, the latter estimated by measurement of epithelial proliferation indices in rectal mucosal biopsies, showed that epithelial proliferation was significantly lower in rural and urban Blacks than in Whites. The diets of all the Black subgroups were characterized by a low animal product and high boiled maize-meal content, whereas Whites consumed more fresh animal products, cheese, and wheat products. Blacks consumed below RDA quantities of fiber (43% of RDA), vitamin A (78%), C (62%), folic acid (80%) and calcium (67%), whereas Whites consumed more animal protein (177% of RDA) and fat (153%). Fasting and food-induced breath methane production was two to three times higher in blacks. It was concluded that the low prevalence of colon cancer in Black Africans cannot be explained by dietary "protective" factors, such as fiber, calcium, vitamins A, C and folic acid, but by the absence of "aggressive" factors, including excess animal protein and fat.[15] On the present hypothesis, the relative absence of vitamin A in the diet is "protective".

Vitamin A deficiency (VAD)

VAD is said to be a major public health problem in more than half of all countries and, along with protein malnutrition, the most common nutritional disorder in the world. It is estimated that approximately 200 million preschool-aged children in developing countries have biochemical VAD and 5 million are clinically affected by the deficiency; that is, based on the prevalence of plasma retinol concentrations below 0.70 μmol/L (or < 20 μg/dl). Other groups of people said to be at high risk for VAD are pregnant and lactating women, and the deficiency is considered endemic in Africa and South-East Asia.[16]

Serum retinol concentrations are lower in people of sub-Saharan Africa and African Americans than in European Americans.[17,18] However, rather than indicating a state of low or deficient vitamin A nutritional status they may instead reflect lower liver stores of vitamin A and/or reduced mobilization and secretion of vitamin A, which may be a characteristic feature of people of West Central African descent, as an evolutionary physiological adaptation to endemic parasitemia. Low serum retinol levels in African Americans could also obscure potentially important but as yet undetermined differences between Africans, African and European Americans on other measures of vitamin nutritional status, notably serum and liver concentrations of retinyl esters and retinoic acid, which are predicted to be higher compared to those of European Americans. New data on these questions may have implications for understanding the overall health status of people of different ancestral origins, for interpreting health disparities, and for international public health interventions to reduce morbidity and mortality rates.

In fact, ongoing vitamin A supplementation programs have become increasingly controversial.[19] Randomly controlled supplementation programs not only showed no reduction in the incidence of diarrhea or respiratory infections but significant increases in respiratory infection rates in children receiving the vitamin A capsules. Detrimental effects on respiratory illnesses were most marked in children with adequate nutritional status.[19,20] A meta-analysis of the impact of capsule programs on child morbidity from diarrhoea and respiratory infections, based on nine randomized controlled trials, found that the combined results indicated no overall protective effect of vitamin A supplementation on the incidence of diarrhea, and slightly increased the incidence of respiratory tract infections.[21] Furthermore, a recent quasi-experimental study and review of the literature on the effect of VAS on anemia and anthropometric failure among children 6–59 months found that all studies "support the findings of this study, that universal periodic doses of VAS may not be useful in preventing anaemia, anthropometric failure, and childhood infections in India".[22]

Slowing the Metabolism of Vitamin A

Genetic diversity is greater in general in Africa than in other continental populations; variability in genes encoding drug metabolizing enzymes may also contribute to the high numbers of adverse drug reactions reported in sub-Saharan Africa.[23,24] The ancestry of African Americans is mainly from Niger-Kordofanian (~ 71%) rather than other African populations;[25] that is, from areas of malaria endemicity. As predicted, African Americans have a lower rate of fat and fatty acid metabolism than European Americans.[26] In one study comparing obese African American and European American in terms of the capacity of skeletal muscle to oxidize fatty acids, oxidizing capacity was 25% lower in African American women than in European American women ($P < 0.05$); mitochondrial and microsomal acyl-CoA synthetase (ACS) were also significantly lower in African American women ($P < 0.005$), suggesting that decreased fatty acid oxidation by skeletal muscle could contribute to the maintenance of obesity.[27]

African Americans also have lower rates of CYP2D6- and CYP2C19-dependent drug metabolism compared to EAs.[28] The cytochrome P450 (CYP) 26 enzymes are specifically involved in the catabolism of retinoic acid (RA) to oxidized metabolites and are highly expressed in the liver, small intestine, and mitochondrial membranes.[29] The availability of RA is regulated by a balance between the synthesizing enzymes (retinaldehyde dehydrogenases-RALDHs) and the catabolizing CYP26 enzymes. While much is known about the function of RALDHs during development, little is known about the role of the CYP26 enzymes, and the differences hypothesized here in metabolism and catabolism between African Americans and European Americans.

In conclusion, data to support the proposed evolutionary adaptations to parasitic diseases are currently limited, but the hypothesized differences between African and European Americans in vitamin A concentrations, tissue locations, and metabolism are readily testable via case-control studies of population groups and organ-specific diseases.

A Note on Diets

The malaria parasite selectively absorbs vitamin A from the host liver, and its use in reproduction has been proposed to contribute to the pathogenesis of the disease. The suggestion is that reduced vitamin A metabolism and catabolism in people of West Central African descent is an evolutionary physiological adaptation to the ancestral environment, causing vitamin A to accumulate and thereby weaken the malaria parasite and reduce disease severity and lethality. In fact, vitamin A is cytotoxic in higher concentration as well as mutagenic and teratogenic and has a direct inhibitory effect on the growth of *Plasmodium falciparum* both in vitro and in vivo.[30]

The mainly plant-based diets of West Central Africa, being low in retinyl esters[31] and high in vitamin A-absorbing fiber, could themselves contribute to health and to an overall state of balance in nutritional status; that is, between the postulated sub-toxic background level of vitamin A in people of West Central African descent, on the one hand and, on the other, the important function of this background state in weakening the malaria parasite and reducing its lethality. Children and teenagers in the US derive >80% of their vitamin A from animal sources and the average adult derives >65%.[32] In Uganda the comparable figures are 5-25% for preschool children and 5-20% for adults.[33]

Other diets evolved in Africa outside areas of malaria endemicity, depending on prevailing conditions and resources. For instance, the Maasai people of Kenya and northern Tanzania are nomadic herdsmen living at a high altitude where mosquitos are typically absent. Their traditional diet consisted mostly of milk, meat, and blood, and little carbohydrate. Yet despite their high fat and cholesterol diet, the Maasai had low blood cholesterol levels, low rates of cholesterol gallstones, low blood pressure, and low rates of atherosclerotic coronary artery disease,[34-36] suggesting a genetic basis for their protection against hypercholesterolemia.

In a search to identify genes under selection in the Maasai related to these unusual dietary pressures, Wagh et al.[37] scanned the genome looking for genetic signatures of natural selection. Based on DNA data collected from groups of people from genetically diverse human populations that included a group of Maasai from Kenya (n=156), the strongest signal of selection was a region of chromosome 2 containing the lactase gene, responsible for breaking down the lactose present in milk.

Lactase persistence, the ability of adults to digest the lactose in milk, varies widely in human populations and represents an adaptation to the domestication of dairying animals and the consumption of their milk.[38]

Another fieldwork study on the Maasai showed that a major contributor to their diet is a high percentage of fermented milk – a kind of yoghurt. The Maasai have strongly sweetened milk tea for breakfast, and some eat a kind of "porridge" in the morning, a liquid mixture of cornmeal, water, milk and sugar. For lunch there will be milk and "Ugali", a kind of polenta made from cornmeal and water. Dinner is similar to lunch.[39]

References

1. Ko Y-H, Wong T-C, Hsu Y-Y, Kuo K-L, Yang SH. The correlation between body fat, visceral fat, and nonalcoholic fatty liver disease. Metabolic Syndrome and Related Disorders 2017; 15:6: 304-311.
2. Saeed A, Dullaart RPF, Schreuder TCMA, Blokzijl H, Faber KN. Disturbed vitamin A metabolism in non-alcoholic fatty liver disease (NAFLD). Nutrients 2017 Dec 29;10(1):29. doi: 10.3390/nu10010029. PMID: 29286303; PMCID: PMC5793257)
3. Hoffman DJ, Wang ZM, Gallagher D et al. Comparison of visceral adipose tissue mass in adult African Americans and whites. Obesity 2013; https://doi.org/10.1038/oby.2005.9
4. Wolf G. Release of stored retinol from adipocytes. Nutr Rev 1998; 56: 29-30.
5. Frey S, Vogel S. Vitamin A metabolism and adipose tissue biology. Nutrients 2011; 3(1):27-39. doi:10.3390/nu3010027
6. Li Y, Wongsiriroj N, Blaner WS. The multifaceted nature of retinoid transport and metabolism. Hepatobiliary Surg Nutr 2014; 3(3):126-139. doi: 10.3978/j.issn.2304-3881.2014.05.04
7. Giaquinto AN, Miller KD, Tossas KY, Winn RA, Jemal A, Siegel RL. Cancer statistics for African American/Black People 2022. CA Cancer J Clin. 2022 May;72(3):202-229. doi: 10.3322/caac.21718

8. David SP, Wang A, Kapphahn K, et al. Gene by Environment Investigation of Incident Lung Cancer Risk in African-Americans. EBioMedicine 2016 Jan 11;4:153-61. doi: 10.1016/j.ebiom.2016.01.002. PMID: 26981579; PMCID: PMC4776066.
9. Blomhoff R, Green MH, Berg T et al. Transport and storage of vitamin A. Science 1990; 250:399-404.
10. Timoneda J, Rodríguez-Fernández L, Zaragozá R et al., Vitamin A deficiency and the lung. Nutrients 2018 Aug 21;10(9):1132. doi: 10.3390/nu10091132. PMID: 30134568; PMCID: PMC6164133.
11. Powell IJ, Meyskens FL Jr. African American men and hereditary/ familial prostate cancer: Intermediate-risk populations for chemoprevention trials. Urology. 2001 Apr;57(4 Suppl 1):178-81. doi: 10.1016/s0090-4295(00)00968-7. PMID: 11295621.
12. Wang Y, Corr JG, Thaler HT, et al: Decreased growth of established human prostate LNCaP tumors in nude mice fed a low-fat diet. J Natl Cancer Inst 87: 1456–1462, 1995.
13. Whittemore AS, Kolonel LN, Wu AH, et al: Prostate cancer in relation to diet, physical activity, and body size in blacks, whites, and Asians in the United States and Canada. J Natl Cancer Inst 87: 652–661, 1995.
14. Heshmat MY, Kaul L, Kovi J, Jackson MA, Jackson AG, Jones GW, Edson M, Enterline JP, Worrell RG, Perry SL. Nutrition and prostate cancer: a case-control study. Prostate. 1985;6(1):7-17. doi: 10.1002/pros.2990060103. PMID: 4038555.
15. O'Keefe SJ, Kidd M, Espitalier-Noel G, Owira P. Rarity of colon cancer in Africans is associated with low animal product consumption, not fiber. Am J Gastroenterol 1999 May;94(5):1373-80. doi: 10.1111/j.1572-0241.1999.01089.x. PMID: 10235221.
16. World Health Organization. Global Prevalence of Vitamin A Deficiency in Populations at Risk 1995–2005. World Health Organization; Geneva, Switzerland: 2009. https://apps.who.int/iris/handle/10665/44110
17. Hanson C, Lyden E, Anderson-Berry A, et al. Status of Retinoids and Carotenoids and Associations with Clinical Outcomes in Maternal-Infant Pairs in Nigeria. Nutrients 2018 Sep 12;10(9):1286. doi: 10.3390/nu10091286. Erratum in: Nutrients. 2019 Feb 13;11(2): PMID: 30213044; PMCID: PMC6165164.
18. Hanson C, Lyden E, Abresch C et al. Serum retinol concentrations, race, and socioeconomic status in women of childbearing age in the United States. Nutrients 2016; 8(8). pii: E508. doi: 0.3390/nu8080508.
19. Latham M. The great vitamin A fiasco. World Nutrition May 2010; 1, 1: 12-45. Also available at: www.wphna.org

20. Grotto I, Mimouni M, Gdalevich, Mimouni, D. Vitamin A supplementation and childhood morbidity from diarrhea and respiratory infections: A meta-analysis. Journal of Pediatrics 2003; 142: 297-304.
21. Dibley JM, SadjiminT, Kjolhede CL, Moulton LH. Vitamin A supplementation fails to reduce incidence of acute respiratory illness and diarrhea in preschool-age Indonesian children. Journal of Nutrition 1996; 126: 434-442.
22. Rai RK. Estimated effect of vitamin A supplementation on anaemia and anthropometric failure of Indian children. Pediatr Res 2022; 91:1263–1271. https://doi.org/10.1038/s41390-022-01969-1
23. Rajman I, Knapp L, Morgan T, Masimirembwa C. African Genetic Diversity: Implications for Cytochrome P450-mediated Drug Metabolism and Drug Development. EBioMedicine 2017; Mar;17:67-74. doi: 10.1016/j.ebiom.2017.02.017. Epub 2017 Feb 20. PMID: 28237373; PMCID: PMC5360579.
24. Mouton, JP, Jobanputra, N, Tatz, G, Cohen, K. Serious adverse drug reactions in sub-Saharan Africa in the era of antiretroviral treatment: A systematic review. Pharmacol Res Perspect. 2021; 9:e00875. https://doi.org/10.1002/prp2.875
25. Tishkoff SA, Reed FA, Friedlaender FR et al. The genetic structure and history of Africans and African Americans. Science 2009; 324:1035–1044.
26. Sharp T, Bell M, Grunwald G et al. Differences in resting metabolic rate between white and African American young adults. Obesity Res 2002; 10(8):726-732.
27. Privette JD, Hickner RC, MacDonald KG et al. Fatty acid oxidation by skeletal muscle homogenates from morbidly obese black and white American women. Metabolism 2003; 52(6):735–738.
28. Aklillu E, Herrlin K, Gustafsson LLet al. Evidence for environmental influence on CYP2D6-catalysed debrisoquine hydroxylation as demonstrated by phenotyping and genotyping of Ethiopians living in Ethiopia or in Sweden. Pharmacogenetics 2002; 12(5):375-83.
29. Napoli JL. Retinoic acid: its biosynthesis and metabolism. Prog Nucleic Acid Res Molec Biol 2000; 63:139-88.
30. Hamzah TS, Skinner-Adams TM, Davis E. In vitro antimalarial activity of retinoids and the influence of selective retinoic acid receptor antagonists Acta Tropica 2003; 87(3):345-353. https://doi.org/10.1016/S0001-706X(03)00119-0
31. Haskell M. The challenge to reach nutritional adequacy for vitamin A: beta carotene bioavailability and conversion – evidence in humans. Am J Clin Nutr 2012; 96(5):1193S-1203S.

32. U.S. Department of Agriculture, 2014. Trends in U.S. Per Capita Consumption of Dairy Products, 1970-2012 https://www.ers.usda.gov/amber-waves/2014/june/trends-in-usper-capita-consumption-of-dairy-products-1970-2012/ (Accessed January 23. 2022).
33. Hotz C, Loechl C, Lubowa A et al. Introduction of β-carotene-rich orange sweet potato in rural Uganda resulted in increased vitamin A intakes among children and women and improved vitamin A status among children. J Nutr 2012;142:1871–80.
34. Mann GV, Shaffer RD, Anderson RS et al. Cardiovascular disease in the Maasai. Journal Atheroscler Res 1964; 4:289–312. http://www.ncbi.nlm.nih.gov/pubmed/14193818
35. Biss K, Ho KJ, Mikkelson B et al. Some unique biologic characteristics of the Maasai of East Africa. N Engl J Med 1971; 284:694–699. DOI:10.1056/NEJM197104012841304 http://www.ncbi.nlm.nih.gov/pubmed/5107799
36. Ho KJ, Biss K, Mikkelson B et al. The Masai of East Africa: some unique biological characteristics. Arch Pathol 1971; 91(5):387-410. http://www.ncbi.nlm.nih.gov/pubmed/4103135
37. Wagh K, Bhatia A, Alexe G et al. Lactase persistence and lipid pathway selection in the Maasai. PLOS One 2012; 7(9):e44751. doi: 10.1371/journal.pone.0044751. PMID: 23028602. https://www.wired.com/2012/09/milk-meat-and-blood-how-diet-drives-natural-selection-in-the-maasai/
38. Securely L, Bon C. On the Evolution of Lactase Persistence in Humans. Annual Review of Genomics and Human Genetics 2017; 18:297-319. https://doi.org/10.1146/annurev-genom-091416-035340
39. Friedrich-Schiller-Universität Jena. "Nomadic people's good health baffle scientists." ScienceDaily. ScienceDaily, 18 May 2010. www.sciencedaily.com/releases/2010/05/100517111910.htm

CHAPTER SEVEN

UNDERSTANDING HEALTH DIFFERENCES AFFECTING AFRICAN AMERICANS

The proposed evolutionary adaptations – sequestering vitamin A to other organs outside the liver, and slowing the metabolism and catabolism of vitamin A, causing it to accumulate to sub-toxic concentrations and weaken the parasite – were apparently successful in the environment of sub-Saharan Africa in reducing the severity and lethality of endemic parasitic infections. However, in the environment of North America they are potentially disadvantageous, for two reasons:

1) Vitamin A-absorbing parasitic organisms are generally lacking, and malaria itself is no longer endemic in the United States.

Before the 1950s, malaria was common throughout the southeastern US. However, the use of mosquito screening in living quarters, improved socioeconomic conditions, environmental management and vector-control efforts during the late 1940s, especially use of the insecticide DDT, succeeded in interrupting malaria transmission.[1] In Africa, endemic malaria and the selective absorption of vitamin A by the merozoites and other vitamin A-absorbing organisms probably contribute to the regulation of vitamin A nutritional status;[2-4] that is, in helping to maintain retinoid concentrations below a critical level of toxicity. Conversely, the absence in North America of Plasmodia species and other vitamin A-absorbing organisms is proposed to contribute to increased risks of many chronic diseases and conditions that are related to vitamin A toxicity. This hypothesis awaits testing. However, apart from having a role in Burkitt's lymphoma, malaria itself is inversely associated with many forms of cancer.[5] For instance, endemic or epidemic malaria is significantly associated with reduced risks of lung, stomach and breast cancer.[6]

Parasitic worms are endemic in sub-Saharan Africa and the most common parasitic infection is schistosomiasis, found mostly in poorer communities lacking access to safe drinking water and adequate sanitation.[7,8] About 120 million people in sub-Saharan Africa were reported as having schistosomiasis-related symptoms in 2000;[9] more recently, a high prevalence of intestinal parasitic infection (up to 90%) was reported in children in some sub-Saharan African countries.[10] Exposure to parasitic worms has long been associated with reduced risks of allergies and autoimmune inflammatory diseases; helminth infections also lower the prevalence of the metabolic syndrome and type 2 diabetes, schistosoma mansoni infection being associated with the most significant positive changes in disease outcomes.[11] Conversely, a decline in exposure to commensal (i.e., nonharmful) bacteria and gastrointestinal helminths has been linked to increased rates of allergic and autoimmune inflammatory disorders in developed countries (the "hygiene hypothesis").[12] Low-grade systemic inflammation is also linked to many aging-related chronic conditions, including cardiovascular disease, dementia, cancer, emphysema, osteoporosis, and macular degeneration, and experimental helminth infection is increasingly promoted as a potential treatment for aging-related chronic diseases, due to its anti-inflammatory effects.[13] For example, helminth-derived products have been suggested as a treatment for NAFLD, which is closely related to obesity, diabetes and metabolic syndrome.[14]

The positive impact of helminth infections on chronic inflammatory diseases is tentatively explained as follows:

- Beta-carotene (precursor for vitamin A) has long been suggested to help prevent cardiovascular disease and cancer, the two leading causes of death in the U.S., in view of the toxicity of vitamin A itself.[15] However, contrary to expectation, supplementation with beta-carotene was found to be associated with increased risks of lung cancer and heart disease in current and former smokers,[16] regardless of the tar or nicotine content of cigarettes smoked.[17] (It should be noted, however, that smoking increases the secretion of retinol-binding protein from the liver.[17A]).
  In patients with breast cancer, antioxidant supplementation with vitamins A, C, and E, carotenoids, and iron before and during treatment was associated with an increased risk of breast cancer recurrence and death.[18] These data, coupled with the known teratogenic effect of vitamin A in utero,[19] suggest that vitamin A may be contributing to cardiovascular disease and many forms of cancer. A common feature of these diseases may be increased concentrations and activity of retinyl esters and retinoic acid.
- A variety of helminths spend part of their life cycle in the gastrointestinal tract and exert beneficial effects on glucose and lipid

metabolism. The literature indicates that enteric nematode infections improve obesity-associated type 2 diabetes and the metabolic syndrome.[20]

- On the vitamin A toxicity hypothesis, parasitic infections reduce the severity of these and other chronic inflammatory diseases by selectively absorbing vitamin A and thereby lowering overall vitamin A concentrations.

In summary, the relative absence of vitamin A-absorbing parasites in North America could contribute to the risks of acute and chronic diseases related to vitamin A, especially in people of sub-Saharan African descent.

2) *African Americans have adopted the same dairy-based diet as that of European Americans.*

Compared to Africans, African Americans consume significantly more protein, meat, saturated fat, cholesterol and vitamin A.[21,22] The 2005 Dietary Guidelines for Americans recommends three servings of dairy foods per day, yet fewer than 7 percent of African Americans actually meet the recommendations and are said to be at risk of nutrient deficits.[23] In spite of the alleged under-consumption of dairy products and its being attributed in part to lactose intolerance in this population, dairy foods are recommended for people with lactose intolerance, to reduce their vulnerability to chronic diseases such as hypertension and diabetes.[24,25]

On the other hand, the United States Department of Agriculture (USDA), the agency responsible for the federal Dietary Guidelines, has recommended the avoidance of high-fat dairy products. This led to a 30-year decline in milk sales and a resulting surplus. In response, the USDA established Dairy Management Incorporated (DMI), which partners with fast food companies to create new high-fat dairy products containing higher than usual amounts of cheese. USDA also partnered with fast food corporations to market and promote the products, such as the award-winning campaign “Got Milk?”.

In her paper, “The unbearable whiteness of milk: food oppression and the USDA”, Andrea Freeman argues that USDA’s efforts to reduce the high-fat milk surplus by selling it to fast food consumers not only imposed health costs on Americans generally but disproportionately harmed low-income African Americans and others living in urban centers dominated by fast food restaurants, by exacerbating already significant health disparities affecting African Americans.[26] Freeman further points out that milk has long enjoyed the reputation of being "nature's perfect food." However, Americans have always had an ambivalent relationship to cow's milk.[27]

The habit of drinking milk began in urban areas in the mid-nineteenth century. Sanitary production was not possible at that time, and opponents claimed that close to 50 percent of children fed milk died as a result. Pasteurization eventually eliminated the dangers of drinking contaminated milk, but new methods of mass production have created other health problems.

While the most common argument in favor of milk consumption is that it is a good source of calcium, helping to build strong bones and prevent osteoporosis, research contradicts these claims. Neither diets high in dairy nor in calcium protect against hip fracture.[28,29] Based on large cohort studies in Sweden (61,433 women and 45,339 men), higher milk consumption was associated with mortality and fractures in women, and with mortality (but not with fracture rate) in men. Positive associations were also found between milk intake and markers for oxidative stress and inflammation.[30]

Our hypothesis, that vitamin A is the critical underlying factor in the diverse adverse effects of dairy, is supported by the observation that consumption of vitamin A from cod liver oil, fortified milk and dairy products is associated with reduced bone density and increased risks of hip fracture.[31] Consumption of dairy food, specifically milk, is also associated with increased risks of being diagnosed with and dying from prostate cancer. The hypothesis that a high intake of calcium could account for the association, possibly by lowering 1,25(OH)2 vitamin D levels, was tested by determining calcium intake in relation to prostate cancer risk using 16 years of follow-up data from the Health Professionals Follow-up Study, a prospective cohort study of 47,750 male health professionals with no history of cancer. Higher calcium intake was associated with advanced and fatal prostate cancer.[32] However, the role of vitamin A was not assessed.

Regarding the impact of reducing exposure to vitamin A in breast milk and in breast tissue via lactation, prolonged breastfeeding is strongly associated with reduced risks of breast cancer. In a meta-analysis of breastfeeding patterns and invasive breast cancer, based on 50,302 cases and almost 97,000 controls from combining 47 epidemiological studies, women with breast cancer had fewer births than the controls (2·2 vs 2·6), fewer parous women with cancer than controls had ever breastfed, their average lifetime duration of breastfeeding was shorter, and the relative risk of breast cancer decreased according with increasing months of breastfeeding (from 6·3 to 2·7 per 100 women by age 70). These data suggested that the incidence of breast cancer in developed countries would be reduced by over 50% if women had the same average number of births and duration of breastfeeding that was prevalent in developing countries until recently. Breastfeeding itself could account for two-thirds of estimated reductions in breast cancer incidence.[33]

Breastfeeding also prevents the progression of gestational diabetes (GDM) to type 2 diabetes. In one study, the effect of lactation on postpartum glucose tolerance was tested by collecting postpartum breastfeeding and oral glucose tolerance test data in 520 women. The prevalence of persistent hyperglycemia was significantly lower in women who breast-fed rather than bottle-fed postpartum (8.2% vs 18.4%, $P<0.001$).[34]

In summary, the absence of vitamin A-absorbing parasites and the adoption of the dairy-based US diet, coupled with the proposed physiological adaptations is proposed to cause vitamin A to accumulate to excess, rendering people of West Central African descent particularly sensitive to vitamin A as a cellular toxin, mutagen, and teratogen. This increased exposure to and the accumulation of vitamin A could explain the increased rates of diseases that were once rare in the original environment. The vitamin A-toxicity hypothesis of the overall health profile of people of West Central African descent is depicted in the figure, below.

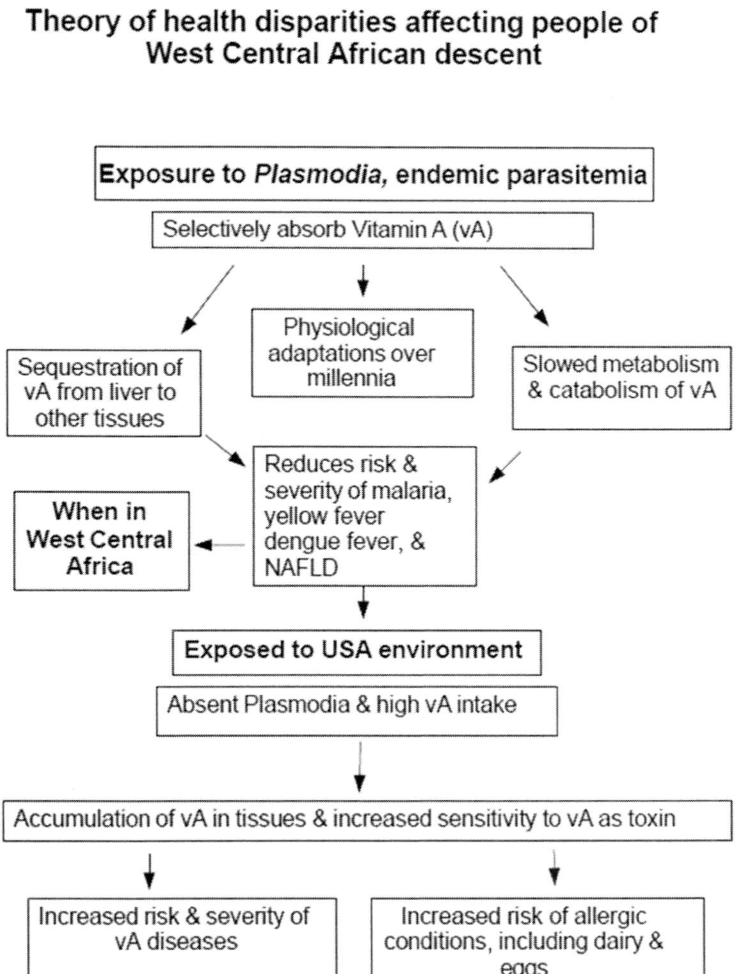

Figure 3. Vitamin A toxicity hypothesis of health disparities affecting people of West Central African descent in the US.

Malaria parasites selectively absorb vitamin A and spend over a week in the liver, the main storage site of vitamin A. Endemic exposure to Plasmodia and other common parasites in the original environment is hypothesized to have led to evolutionary adaptations involving 1) the sequestration of vitamin A from the liver to subcutaneous adipose and other tissues, to reduce its accessibility to the parasite; and 2) reduced vitamin A enzymatic metabolism and catabolism, causing it to accumulate to sub-toxic concentrations and weaken the parasite, thereby reducing the risk of severe disease. These adaptations may have reduced the severity of malaria, yellow fever, dengue, and the risk of NAFLD in people of West Central African descent. However, in North America, where major parasites are absent and high vitamin A-containing diets are the norm, these adaptations may cause vitamin A to accumulate in the tissues, thereby increasing the risk and severity of many chronic diseases. They may also have led to an enhanced sensitivity to vitamin A as a cellular toxin, and increased risks of allergy. These adaptations may be contributing to the emergence of a similar health profile in West Central Africans as western diets are increasingly adopted.

References

1. Andrews JM, Quinby GE, Langmuir AD. Malaria eradication in the United States. American Journal of Public Health 1950; 40:1405–1411.
2. Mizuno Y, Kawazu SI, Kano S et al. In-vitro uptake of vitamin A by Plasmodium falciparum. Annals Trop Med Parasitol 2003; 97:237–43.
3. Stoltzfus RJ, Jalal F, Harvey PW et al. Interactions between vitamin A deficiency and Plasmodium berghei infection in the rat. J Nutr 1989 Dec;119(12):2030-7. doi: 10.1093/jn/119.12.2030. PMID: 2695606.
4. SanJoaquin MA, Molyneux ME. Malaria and vitamin A deficiency in African children: a vicious circle? Malaria J 2009; 8, 134. https://doi.org/10.1186/1475-2875-8-134.
5. Ellis T, Eze E, Raimi-AbrahamT. Malaria and Cancer: a critical review on the established associations and new perspectives. Infect Agent Cancer. 2021 May 13;16(1):33. doi: 10.1186/s13027-021-00370-7. PMID: 33985540; PMCID: PMC8117320.
6. Qin L, Chen C, Chen L, Xue R, Ou-Yang M, Zhou C, Zhao S, He Z, Xia Y, He J, Liu P, Zhong N, Chen X. Worldwide malaria incidence and cancer mortality are inversely associated. Infect Agent Cancer. 2017 Feb 14;12:14. doi: 10.1186/s13027-017-0117-x. PMID: 28228842; PMCID: PMC5307699.
7. WHO. Schistosomiasis (Bilharzia). WHO Regional Office for Africa https://www.afro.who.int/health-topics/schistosomiasis-bilharzia (Accessed December 29, 2022)
8. Mitra AK, Mawson AR. Neglected tropical diseases: epidemiology and global burden. Tropical Medicine and Infectious Disease 2017; 2(3):36. https://doi.org/10.3390/tropicalmed2030036.

9. Chitsulo L, Engels D, Montresor A, Savioli L. The global status of schistosomiasis and its control. Acta Trop 2000; 77:41-51).
10. Hailegebriel T. Prevalence of intestinal parasitic infections and associated risk factors among students at Dona Berber primary school, Bahir Dar, Ethiopia. BMC Infect Dis 2017; 17:362. https://doi.org/10.1186/s12879-017-2466-x
11. Rennie C, Fernandez R, Donnelly S, McGrath KC. The impact of helminth infection on the incidence of metabolic syndrome: a systematic review and meta-analysis. Front Endocrinol (Lausanne). 2021 Aug 12;12:728396. doi: 10.3389/fendo.2021.728396. PMID: 34456879; PMCID: PMC8397462.
12. Strachan DP. Hay fever, hygiene and household size. BMJ 1989; 299:1259–60.
13. Zhang B, Gems D. Gross ways to live long: Parasitic worms as an anti-inflammaging therapy? eLife 2021; 10:e65180. https://doi.org/10.7554/eLife.65180).
14. Liu X, Jiang Y, Ye J, Wang X. Helminth infection and helminth-derived products: A novel therapeutic option for non-alcoholic fatty liver disease. Front Immunol. 2022 Oct 3;13:999412. doi: 10.3389/fimmu.2022.999412.
15. Peto R, Doll R, Buckley J. et al. Can dietary beta-carotene materially reduce human cancer rates? Nature 1981; 290, 201–208. https://doi.org/10.1038/290201a0).
16. O'Connor EA, Evans CV, Ivlev I, et al. Vitamin and Mineral Supplements for the Primary Prevention of Cardiovascular Disease and Cancer: Updated Evidence Report and Systematic Review for the US Preventive Services Task Force. JAMA. 2022;327(23):2334–2347. doi:10.1001/jama.2021.15650.
17. Middha P, Weinstein SJ, Männistö S, Albanes D, Mondul AM. β-Carotene supplementation and lung cancer incidence in the Alpha-Tocopherol, Beta-Carotene Cancer Prevention Study: The role of tar and nicotine. Nicotine Tob Res 2019 Jul 17;21(8):1045-1050. doi: 10.1093/ntr/nty115. PMID: 29889248; PMCID: PMC6636175.
17A. Gao S, Wang Y-H, Li M. Cigarette smoking increases levels of retinol-binding protein-4 in healthy men with normal glucose tolerance. Chinese Medical Journal 2012; 125(10):1686-1689. https://pubmed.ncbi.nlm.nih.gov/22800884/
18. Ambrosone CB, Zirpoli GR, Hutson AD et al. Dietary supplement use during chemotherapy and survival outcomes of patients with breast cancer enrolled in a cooperative group clinical trial (SWOG S0221). J

Clin Oncol 2020 Mar 10;38(8):804-814. Doi:10.1200/JCO.19.01203. Epub 2019 Dec 19.
19. Jordan, R. Vitamin A, its congeners, and neural tube defects: their mutagenic effects on the developing fetus during embryogenesis. Nutrition Noteworthy 1998; 1(1). Retrieved from https://escholarship.org/uc/item/8jn036ph
20. Shea-Donohue T, Qin B, Smith A. Parasites, nutrition, immune responses and biology of metabolic tissues. Parasite Immunol 2017 May;39(5):10.1111/pim.12422. doi: 10.1111/pim.12422. Epub 2017 Mar 22. PMID: 28235148; PMCID: PMC5863236.
21. Li W, Youssef G, Procter-Gray E, Olendzki B, Cornish T, Hayes R, Churchill L, Kane K, Brown K, Magee MF. Racial Differences in Eating Patterns and Food Purchasing Behaviors among Urban Older Women. J Nutr Health Aging. 2017;21(10):1190-1199. doi: 10.1007/s12603-016-0834-7. PMID: 29188879; PMCID: PMC5726305.
22. O'Keefe SJ, Chung D, Mahmoud N et al. Why do African Americans get more colon cancer than Native Africans? J Nutr 2007 Jan;137(1 Suppl):175S-182S. doi: 10.1093/jn/137.1.175S.
23. Beydoun MA, Gary TL, Caballero H, Lawrence RS, Cheskin LJ, Wang Y. Ethnic differences in dairy and related nutrient consumption among US adults and their associations with obesity, central obesity, and the metabolic syndrome. American Journal of Clinical Nutrition 2008; 87:1914-25.
24. National Medical Association. Lactose Intolerance and African Americans: Implications for the Consumption of Appropriate Intake Levels of Key Nutrients. J Nat Med Assoc. Supplement to October 2009; Volume 101, No. 10.
25. National Dairy Council. Dairy's Role in African-American Health: Benefits Beyond Bone Health https://efnep.ucanr.edu/files/101690.pdf Accessed January 3, 2023.
26. Freeman A. The unbearable whiteness of milk: food oppression and the USDA. UC IRVINE LAW REVIEW 2013; Vol. 3:1251. Available at: https://scholarship.law.uci.edu/ucilr/vol3/iss4/16,
27. Dupuis ME. Nature's perfect food: How milk became America's drink. New York University Press, United States, 2002.
28. Feskanich D, Willett WC, Stampfer MJ, Colditz GA. Milk, dietary calcium, and bone fractures in women: a 12-year prospective study. Am J Public Health. 1997 Jun;87(6):992-7. doi: 10.2105/ajph.87.6.992. PMID: 9224182; PMCID: PMC1380936.

29. Owusu W, Willett WC, Feskanich D et al. Calcium intake and the incidence of forearm and hip fractures among men. Journal of Nutrition 1997; 127(9):1782–1787. https://doi.org/10.1093/jn/127.9.1782.
30. Michaëlsson K, Wolk A, Langenskiöld S, Basu S et al. Milk intake and risk of mortality and fractures in women and men: cohort studies. BMJ 2014 Oct 28;349:g6015. doi: 10.1136/bmj.g6015. PMID: 25352269; PMCID: PMC4212225.)
31. Melhus H, Michaëlsson K, Kindmark A, Bergström R et al. Excessive dietary intake of vitamin A is associated with reduced bone mineral density and increased risk for hip fracture. Ann Intern Med 1998 Nov 15;129(10):770-8. doi: 10.7326/0003-4819-129-10-199811150-00003)
32. Giovannucci W, Liu Y, Stampfer MJ, Willett WC. A prospective study of calcium intake and incident and fatal prostate cancer. Cancer Epidemiol Biomarkers Prev. 2006; 15(2):203–210. https://doi.org/10.1158/1055-9965.EPI-05-0586 .)
33. WHO Collaborative Group on Hormonal Factors in Breast Cancer. Breast cancer and breastfeeding: collaborative reanalysis of individual data from 47 epidemiological studies in 30 countries, including 50,302 women with breast cancer and 96,973 women without the disease. Lancet 2002; 360 (9328):187-195. DOI: https://doi.org/10.1016/S0140-6736(02)09454-0
34. O'Reilly MW, Avalos G, Dennedy MC, O'Sullivan EP, Dunne F. Atlantic DIP: high prevalence of abnormal glucose tolerance post partum is reduced by breast-feeding in women with prior gestational diabetes mellitus. Eur J Endocrinol. 2011 Dec;165(6):953-9. doi: 10.1530/EJE-11-0663. Epub 2011 Sep 21. PMID: 21937504.

CHAPTER EIGHT

DISPARITIES INVOLVING ORGAN-SPECIFIC DISEASES

Rates of colorectal cancer in African Americans are dramatically higher than in Africans (60/100,000 vs <1/100,000), and slightly higher than in European Americans.[1] African Americans also have higher death rates from cancer of the breast, cervix, ovary and lung, and a twofold higher rate of triple-negative breast cancer, a more aggressive type.[2]

Breast cancer incidence is higher overall in women of European descent than in women of African ancestry, but African Americans are more likely to be diagnosed before age 40 and to have breast tumors with more aggressive features, including high-grade and negative estrogen receptor status.[3] Higher dairy milk consumption is also associated with a 50 percent increased risk of breast cancer, although current nutritional guidelines recommend it.[4] As noted in Chapter 7, reducing exposure to vitamin A in breast milk and in breast tissue through prolonged breastfeeding is strongly associated with reduced risks of breast cancer, the relative risk of breast cancer decreasing with increasing months of breastfeeding.[5] However, apparently at odds with the vitamin A toxicity hypothesis, the first study of the association between vitamin A dietary intake risk of breast cancer in African Americans reported an inverse association of total vitamin A intake and estrogen-receptor-positive breast cancer. This was an analysis of data from 3564 cancer cases and 11,843 controls in the African American Breast Cancer Epidemiology and Risk (AMBER) Consortium.[6] Interestingly, the association was significant among premenopausal but not postmenopausal women, although the disease is more common in the latter,[7] suggesting that factors related to breast tumor biology could explain the conundrum.

African American males in 2014 also had the highest incidence rate of prostate cancer and were more likely to die of the disease than any other group.[8] Consistent with the overall model presented here, the risk factors for prostate cancer include high dietary intakes of vitamin A.[9]

The death rate for all cancers combined is 25 percent higher for African Americans than for European Americans.[10] African Americans also have the highest death rates from stroke[11] and are twice as likely to develop

Alzheimer's disease and other dementias as European Americans,[12] possibly related to increased concentrations of vitamin A in the brain.

African Americans, having a higher percentage of abdominal subcutaneous adipose tissue and a lower percentage of abdominal visceral fat,[13,14] also have lower rates of NAFLD than those of other ethnic groups,[15] and significantly lower triglyceride levels than Hispanic and European Americans.[16] These differences in disease rates may be related to increased concentrations and expression of retinoids in the organs in question in African Americans compared to European Americans, and increased accumulation due to reduced metabolism and catabolism. Yet African Americans who do develop NAFLD are overrepresented in terms of disease precursors to CVD, including obesity, hypertension, and diabetes, and are more prone than European Americans to develop advanced liver disease.

In the Jackson Heart Study, a cohort of over 5,000 older African Americans, participants with high levels of abdominal visceral and liver fat had high rates of hypertension, diabetes, and dyslipidemia.[17] Fatty liver was also associated with coronary atherosclerotic calcification independent of abdominal visceral fat or Body Mass Index.[18] Other studies indicate a strong association between NAFLD and atherosclerotic calcification.[19]

Growing evidence implicates retinoids in the fundamental processes relevant to atherosclerosis, including vascular calcification and endothelial dysfunction. Mice fed excess vitamin A for 12 months developed heart valve stenosis and leaflet calcification, suggesting that hypervitaminosis A is a risk factor for calcific aortic valve disease.[20] The effects of retinoids on lipid metabolism and adipogenesis may indirectly cause inflammation and atherosclerosis.[21] However, African Americans are typically less likely to develop coronary atherosclerotic calcification and have markedly lower levels than European Americans when they do develop it,[22] possibly related to their low risk of osteoporosis, higher bone densities, and lower bone turnover rates.[23]

What could explain the paradoxical observations that African Americans are at increased risk of metabolic syndrome despite lower levels of liver fat, and prone to advanced liver disease? The postulated tendency toward reduced vitamin A metabolism and hence increased vitamin A accumulation could account for these facts. Even with lower levels of liver fat, African Americans may be more sensitive to vitamin A as a toxin and more likely to experience inflammatory changes, e.g., in the liver, indicated by increased liver enzymes, as well as more prone to obesity, hypertension, and diabetes and to severe manifestations and the secondary consequences of these conditions.

In partial support of this hypothesis, a 12-year prospective study of liver enzymes and diabetes risk in the Atherosclerosis Risk in Communities (ARIC) study, involving 7,495 European and 1,842 African Americans without diabetes, found that high liver enzyme levels were independently associated with diabetes risk. The enzyme gamma-glutamyl transferase (GGT) was most strongly associated with diabetes, even at levels considered within the normal range (≤60 U/l). Adjusted incidence rates of diabetes by quartiles of liver enzymes were similar in terms of gender but higher in African Americans. These findings have suggested that abnormal liver enzymes precede the diagnosis of diabetes by many years and that individuals with elevated liver enzymes, even within supposedly normal limits, are at high risk for diabetes, especially African Americans.[24] In summary, the increased susceptibility of people of West Central African descent to certain chronic diseases, including diabetes, from which they were originally protected, may be due to the adoption of vitamin A-rich North American diets and to an increased sensitivity to vitamin A as a toxin, resulting from its slower metabolism and catabolism and greater accumulation.

Of special interest is the observation that widening disparities in heart disease mortality rates have occurred only since the 1970s. In Mississippi before that time, available records suggest that differences in cardiovascular disease (CVD) death rates between African and European Americans were less marked or even nonexistent. [According to the 2019 U.S. Census estimates, African Americans accounted for 37.8% of the state's population, the highest in the nation.[25]] African Americans had similar CVD rates to those of European American Mississippians and Americans in general, and African American males had lower CVD death rates than either white Mississippi males or white US males.[26]

It was in the 1980s that the magnitude of the disparity between African and European Americans in CVD mortality rates increased dramatically. Yet during that time, race-linked factors such as discrimination and limited access to health care were either static or improving. Other factors to consider include changes in occupational opportunities as well as dietary influences favoring processed and fast-food consumption;[27] these include foods fortified by or supplemented with vitamin A. Cheese consumption has increased in recent decades, as has vitamin A-fortified low-fat milk. Cheese availability (used as a measure of consumption) was 11.4 lbs in 1970 compared to 33.5 lbs/person in 2012, nearly three times higher than the earlier rate. Consumption of frozen pizza, macaroni and cheese, and pre-packaged cheese has also increased.[28] (see Figure 4).

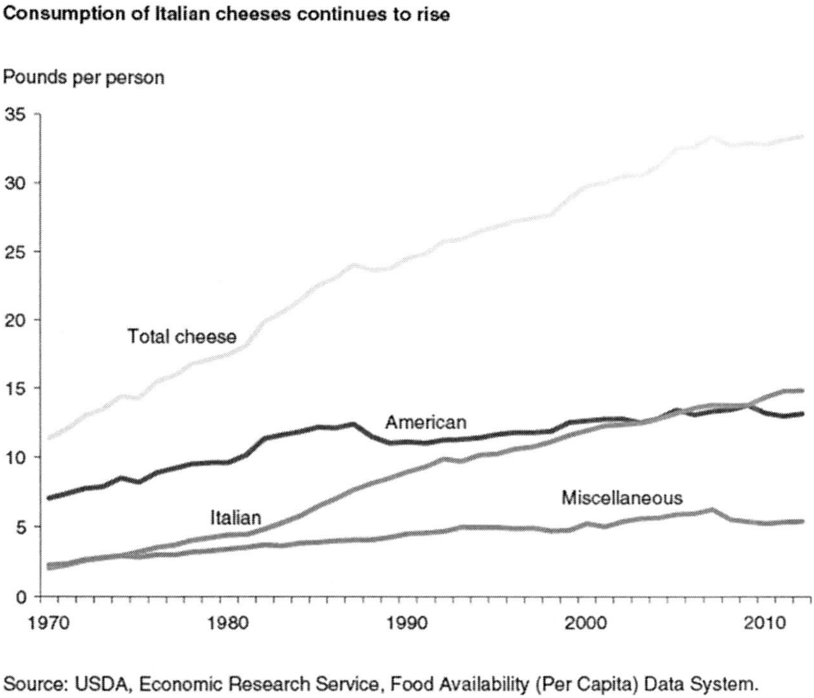

Figure 4. Consumption of cheese in the United States, 1970-2010

In 1908, it was observed that rabbits fed meat, milk and eggs developed arterial lesions like those of atherosclerosis in humans.[29] The association between dairy consumption and heart disease-related clinical outcomes remains controversial,[30] partly because the traditional focus on fat, cholesterol and calcium as risk factors may have obscured the role of vitamin A itself. Research is needed to assess vitamin A intake directly, including food and vitamin supplements, to determine its association with the many disparities in health outcomes affecting African Americans compared to European Americans and other groups.

References

1. Williams R, White P, Nieto J et al. Colorectal cancer in African Americans: an update, prepared by the Committee on Minority Affairs and Cultural Diversity, American College of Gastroenterology. Clin Trans Gastroenterol 2016; 7(7), e185.

2. Pickle LW, Mungiole M, Jones GK et al. Atlas of United States mortality – National Center for Health Statistics (U.S.), Centers for Disease Control and Prevention, Hyattsville, Maryland. December 1996. DHHS Publication No. (PHS) 97-1015. https://www.cdc.gov/nchs/data/misc/atlasres.pdf
3. Amend K, Hicks D, Ambrosone CB. Breast cancer in African-American women: differences in tumor biology from European-American women. Cancer Research 2006; 66(17):8327–8330.)
4. Fraser GE, Jaceldo-Siegl K, Orlich M et al. Dairy, soy, and risk of breast cancer: those confounded milks. Int J Epidemiol 2020; 49(5):1526–1537, https://doi.org/10.1093/ije/dyaa007.
5. WHO Collaborative Group on Hormonal Factors in Breast Cancer. Breast cancer and breastfeeding: collaborative reanalysis of individual data from 47 epidemiological studies in 30 countries, including 50,302 women with breast cancer and 96,973 women without the disease. Lancet 2002; 360 (9328):187-195. DOI: https://doi.org/10.1016/S0140-6736(02)09454-0.
6. Bitsie KR, Cheng TYD, McCann SE, Zirpoli G. et al. Dietary vitamin A and breast cancer risk in black women: The African American Breast Cancer Epidemiology and Risk (AMBER) Consortium. The Journal of Nutrition 2021; 51(12):3725–3737, https://doi.org/10.1093/jn/nxab278.
7. Kwan ML, Kushi LH, Weltzien E, Maring B, Kutner SE, Fulton RS, et al. Epidemiology of breast cancer subtypes in two prospective cohort studies of breast cancer survivors. Breast Cancer Res 2009; 11:R31. https://doi.org/10.1186/bcr2261
8. CDC. Prostate Cancer Rates by Race and Ethnicity, 2018 https://www.cdc.gov/cancer/prostate/statistics/race.htm
9. Hanks GE, Myers CE, Scardino PT. Chapter 35: Cancer of the prostate. In DeVita VT Jr., Hellman S, Rosenberg SA, eds. Cancer: Principles and practice of oncology. Philadelphia: J.B. Lippincott Company, 1993:1073-1113.
10. American Cancer Society, 2018. https://www.cancer.gov/aboutnci/organization/crchd/cancer-health-disparities-fact-sheet (Accessed January 23, 2022).
11. CDC, Stroke. 2018 https://www.cdc.gov/nchs/data/misc/atlasres.pdf
12. Barnes LL, Bennett DA. Alzheimer's disease In African Americans: risk factors and challenges for the future. Health Affairs (Project Hope) 2014; 33(4):580–586.
13. De Lucia Rolfe E, Ong KK, Sleigh A et al. Abdominal fat depots associated with insulin resistance and metabolic syndrome risk factors in black African young adults. BMC Public Health 2015; 15, 1013.

https://doi.org/10.1186/s12889-015-2147-x
14. Rønn PF, Andersen GS, Lauritzen T, et al. Abdominal visceral and subcutaneous adipose tissue and associations with cardiometabolic risk in Inuit, Africans and Europeans: a cross-sectional study. BMJ Open 2020;10:e038071. doi: 10.1136/bmjopen-2020-038071.
15. Bonacini M, Kassamali F, Kari S, Lopez Barrera N, Kohla M. Racial differences in prevalence and severity of non-alcoholic fatty liver disease. World J Hepatol. 2021 Jul 27;13(7):763-773. doi: 10.4254/wjh.v13.i7.763. PMID: 34367497; PMCID: PMC8326166.
16. Foster T, Anania FA, Li D, Katz R, Budoff M. The prevalence and clinical correlates of nonalcoholic fatty liver disease (NAFLD) in African Americans: the multiethnic study of atherosclerosis (MESA). Dig Dis Sci 2013; 58(8):2392-8. doi: 10.1007/s10620-013-2652-7.
17. Liu J, Fox CS, Hickson D, et al. Fatty liver, abdominal visceral fat, and cardiometabolic risk factors: the Jackson Heart Study. Arterioscler Thromb Vasc Biol 2011; 31(11):2715-22. doi: 10.1161/ATVBAHA.111.234062.
18. Liu J, Musani SK, Bidulescu A et al. Fatty liver, abdominal adipose tissue and atherosclerotic calcification in African Americans: the Jackson Heart Study. Atherosclerosis 2012; 224(2):521-5. doi: 10.1016/j.atherosclerosis.2012.07.042.
19. Lee JE, Lee YJ, Chung SY et al. Severity of nonalcoholic fatty liver disease is associated with subclinical cerebro-cardiovascular atherosclerosis risk in Korean men. PLoS One 2018; 13(3):e0193191. doi: 10.1371/journal.pone.0193191. eCollection 2018.
20. Huk DJ, Hammond HL, Kegechika H et al. Increased dietary intake of vitamin A promotes aortic valve calcification in vivo. Arterioscler Thromb Vasc Biol. 2013 Feb;33(2):285-93. doi: 10.1161/ATVBAHA.112.300388.
21. Rhee EJ, Nallamshetty S, Plutzky J. Retinoid metabolism and its effects on the vasculature. Biochim Biophys Acta 2012; 1821(1):230-40. doi: 10.1016/j.bbalip.2011.07.001.
22. Divers J, Palmer ND, Langefeld CD et al. Genome-wide association study of coronary artery calcified atherosclerotic plaque in African Americans with type 2 diabetes. BMC Genet 2017; 18(1):105. doi: 10.1186/s12863-017-0572-9.
23. Overfield T. Biological variation in health and illness: Race, age and sex differences.
2nd Edition. CRC Press, Boca Raton, FL. 1995.

24. Schneider AL, Lazo M, Ndumele CE et al. Liver enzymes, race, gender and diabetes risk: the Atherosclerosis Risk in Communities (ARIC) Study. Diabet Med 2013; 30(8):926-33. doi: 10.1111/dme.12187.
25. U.S. Census Bureau Quick Facts: Mississippi. https://www.census.gov/quickfacts/MS (Accessed January 9, 2023).
26. Jones DW, Sempos CT, Thom TJ et al. Rising levels of cardiovascular mortality in Mississippi, 1979-1995. Am J Med Sci 2000; 319(3):131-7.
27. Cosby AG, Brown L, Taylor T et al. An assessment of cardiovascular health in Mississippi: A focus on racial disparities in mortality, behavioral risk factors, and knowledge. Social Science Research Center, Mississippi State University. March 2006. http://www.ssrc.msstate.edu
28. USDA. US Department of Agriculture, 2014. Trends in U.S. Per Capita Consumption of Dairy Products, 1970-2012 https://www.ers.usda.gov/amber-waves/2014/june/trends-inus-per-capita-consumption-of-dairy-products-1970-2012/
29. Ignatovski AI. Influence of animal foods on the organism of rabbits. Izv Imp Voyenno-Med Akad Peter 1908; 16:154-176.
30. Drouin-Chartier JP, Brassard D et al. Systematic review of the association between dairy product consumption and risk of cardiovascular-related clinical outcomes. Adv Nutr 2016;7(6):1026-1040. doi: 10.3945/an.115.011403.

CHAPTER NINE

SENSITIVITY TO VITAMIN A AND RISKS OF ALLERGIES

Allergic diseases are among the most common types of disease and represent a substantial burden on patient functioning and wellbeing; they include rhinitis, asthma, atopic dermatitis, gastrointestinal conditions and food allergies, and tend to aggregate in the same individual.[1] Allergic diseases also disproportionately affect African Americans compared to European Americans. A recent monograph on the subject, *Health Disparities in Allergic Diseases: An Evidence-Based Look at Causes, Conditions, and Outcomes,*[2] addresses important differences in the presentation of the spectrum of allergic diseases worldwide. The review begins: "With the current attention on systemic racism and structural violence in the United States, this book serves as a timely reminder of how racial and socioeconomic disparities play a role in the manifestation of disease. Allergic diseases, as chronic illnesses that often start in childhood and in which severity is most related to the quality of routine healthcare maintenance and health literacy, are a compelling lens in which to view and discuss the power of social determinants of health".[3]

To summarize the thesis presented in this book, health differences affecting people of sub-Saharan African descent in the United States have arisen in part from 1) evolutionary physiological adaptations to challenges in the ancestral environment – in particular the use by parasitic organisms of vitamin A, selectively absorbed from the host for reproduction; and 2) the relative absence of such organisms in North America, coupled with the adoption of dairy-based diets, which have contributed to increases in sensitivity of vitamin A as a toxin and to increasing risks of vitamin A-associated diseases.

On the vitamin A toxicity hypothesis, higher rates of atopy – that is, atopic dermatitis (eczema), other forms of pruritus, and asthma – among African Americans compared to European Americans[4] are due to the proposed evolutionary adaptations: sequestration of vitamin A away from the liver, leading to increased concentrations of vitamin A in the skin and lung; to reduced rates of vitamin A metabolism, inducing vitamin A accumulation and greater sensitivity to it as a toxin; and exposure to the characteristic microbiological and nutritional environment of North America.

Consistent with the hypothesis, the most common adverse effect of topical retinoids is skin irritation, resulting in itching, redness and peeling.[5] Use of therapeutic retinoids is frequently linked to irritant contact dermatitis,[6] and topical retinoid use for skin of color in particular is associated with contact dermatitis, leading to increased risks of post-inflammatory keloid or hypertrophic scarring, and recommendations to start at a lower concentration and titrate upwards.[7] Use of the synthetic retinoid isotretinoin by African American patients with recalcitrant nodulocystic acne was reportedly associated with an early onset flare in areas of the face that were devoid of lesions prior to treatment.[8]

In a birth cohort study of allergic disorders in the Detroit metropolitan area, participants at two years of age were skin tested on a range of potential allergens and their parents were interviewed about wheezing and allergy symptoms. African American children were more likely than White children to have experienced any of the outcomes examined, indicating that disparities in allergic disease outcomes emerge as early as age 2.[9] African Americans are likewise disproportionately burdened by chronic pruritic disorders, including atopic dermatitis, prurigo nodularis, and inflammatory scalp dermatoses.[10]

Stevens-Johnson syndrome (SJS) and the more severe toxic epidermal necrolysis (TEN) are drug-induced conditions forming a continuum of life-threatening disease. Nationally representative inpatient data indicate that African Americans have a substantially higher risk of SJS/TEN than whites in the US population, the drug allopurinol in particular being implicated.[10A]

In a study of food-allergen sensitization in early childhood related to self-identified race or genetic ancestry, 1104 children (mean age: 2.7 years) from an urban multiethnic birth cohort were tested for food sensitization, defined as immunoglobulin E (IgE) levels of $\geq$ 0.35 kilo-units of allergen (kUA)/L, for any of 8 common food allergens. Both self-reported "black race" and African ancestry were associated with food sensitization and with a high number ($\geq$ 3) of food sensitizations. African ancestry was also associated with egg and peanut sensitization.[11]

Retinoid toxicity is linked to bronchial asthma.[12-14] Intakes of vitamin A $\geq$2.5 times the recommended daily amount during pregnancy were associated with increased risks of asthma in school-age children in Norway. Most mothers used cod liver oil, in which the median intake of supplemented vitamin A was $\geq$300 μg/d compared to the standard daily dose of 250 μg.[15]

African Americans are hypothesized to be more sensitive to vitamin A as a toxin than European Americans, associated with higher concentrations of vitamin A in affected tissues. Higher rates of allergic reactions to milk[16] and eggs are also reported in Africans and African Americans compared to European Americans,[17] and 70%-80% of African Americans are lactose intolerant.[18] Cow milk is the most common cause of food allergy and food intolerance in the United States, especially affecting young children.[19] The high content of vitamin A in eggs and in dairy products such as milk and cheese[20] could explain the disparities in question.

Lower rates of alcohol use among African compared to European Americans[21] may reflect the fact that alcohol increases the secretion of vitamin A from the liver and enhances its toxicity.[22]

In a study comparing differences in allergy according to ancestral origins, African Americans had significantly higher odds of allergy to finfish and shellfish compared to European American children as well as higher adjusted odds of asthma.[23] Consistent with the hypothesis, concentrations of preformed vitamin A are highest in fish as well as liver, eggs, and dairy products.[24]

References

1. Pinart M, Albang R, Maier D, Duran-Tauleria E et al. Systematic review on the definition of allergic diseases in children: The MeDALL Study. Int Arch Allergy Immunol 2015; 168(2):110-21. doi: 10.1159/000442414.
2. Mahdavinia M, editor. Health Disparities in Allergic Diseases: An Evidence-Based Look at Causes, Conditions, and Outcomes. 2020. Springer Nature Switzerland AG. ISBN: (Paperback) 978-3030312213.
3. Zheng M. Health disparities in allergic diseases: An evidence-based look at causes, conditions, and outcomes. Yale J Biol Med 2020 Dec 29;93(5):769. PMCID: PMC7757068.
4. Gupta J, Johansson E, Bernstein JA et al. Resolving the etiology of atopic disorders by using genetic analysis of racial ancestry. J Allergy Clin Immunol 2016; 138(3):676-699. doi: 10.1016/j.jaci.2016.02.045.
5. Olson JM, Ameer MA, Goyal A. Vitamin A toxicity. [Updated 2022 Aug 8]. In: StatPearls [Internet]. Treasure Island (FL): StatPearls Publishing; 2022.
https://www.ncbi.nlm.nih.gov/books/NBK532916/#_NBK532916_pubdet

6. Veraldi S, Brena M, Barbareschi M. Allergic contact dermatitis caused by topical antiacne drugs. Expert Rev Clin Pharmacol 2015; 8(4):377-81. doi: 10.1586/17512433.2015.1046839.
7. Davis EC, Callender VD. A review of acne in ethnic skin: Pathogenesis, clinical manifestations, and management strategies. J Clin Aesthetic Dermatol 2010; 3(4):24-38.
8. Kelly AP, Sampson DD. Recalcitrant nodulocystic acne in black Americans: treatment with isotretinoin. J Nat Med Assoc 1987; 79:1266-70.
9. Wegienka G, Havstad S, Joseph CL, Zoratti E et al. Racial disparities in allergic outcomes in African Americans emerge as early as age 2 years. Clin Exp Allergy 2012 Jun;42(6):909-17. doi: 10.1111/j.1365-2222.2011.03946.x. PMID: 22909162; PMCID: PMC3428737.
10. Ingrasci G, El-Kashlan N, Alexis A, Yosipovitch G. Chronic itch in African Americans: an unmet need. Arch Dermatol Res 2022 Jul;314(5):405-415. doi: 10.1007/s00403-021-02255-6.
11. A. Lu N, Rai SK, Terkeltaub R, Kim SC, Menendez ME, Choi HK. Racial disparities in the risk of Stevens-Johnson Syndrome and toxic epidermal necrolysis as urate-lowering drug adverse events in the United States. Semin Arthritis Rheum. 2016 Oct;46(2):253-258. doi: 10.1016/j.semarthrit.2016.03.014.
12. Kumar R, Tsai HJ, Hong X, Liu X, et al. Race, ancestry, and development of food-allergen sensitization in early childhood. Pediatrics. 2011 Oct;128(4):e821-9. doi: 10.1542/peds.2011-0691. Epub 2011 Sep 2. PMID: 21890831; PMCID: PMC3182844.).
13. Mawson AR. Could bronchial asthma be an endogenous, pulmonary expression of retinoid intoxication? Front Biosci 2001; 6:D973-85.
14. Solt LA, Griffin PR, Burris TP. Ligand regulation of retinoic acid receptor-related orphan receptors: implications for development of novel therapeutics. Curr Opin Lipidol 2010; 21(3):204-11. doi: 10.1097/MOL.0b013e328338ca18.
15. Na H, Lim H, Choi G et al. Concomitant suppression of TH2 and TH17 cell responses in allergic asthma by targeting retinoic acid receptor-related orphan receptor γt. J Allergy Clin Immunol 2017; pii: S0091-6749(17)31481-1. doi: 10.1016/j.jaci.2017.07.050.
16. Parr CL, Magnus MC, Karlstad Ø et al. Vitamin A and D intake in pregnancy, infant supplementation, and asthma development: the Norwegian Mother and Child Cohort. Am J Clin Nutr 2018; 0:1-10, https://doi.org/10.1093/ajcn/nqy016

17. Bailey R, Fileti C, Keith J et al. Lactose intolerance and health disparities among African Americans and Hispanic Americans: An updated consensus statement. J Natl Med Assoc 2013; 105(2): 112-127.
18. Gray CL, Levin ME, du Toit G. Egg sensitization, allergy and component patterns in African children with atopic dermatitis. Pediatr Allergy Immunol 2016; 27(7):709-715. doi:10.1111/pai.12615.
19. National Institute of Diabetes and Digestive and Kidney Diseases. National Institutes of Health, Washington, DC. 2009. http://digestive.niddk.nih.gov/ddiseases/pubs/lactoseintolerance/
20. Manuyakorn W, Tanpowpong P. Cow milk protein allergy and other common food allergies and intolerances. Paediatr Int Child Health. 2019 Feb;39(1):32-40. doi: 10.1080/20469047.2018.1490099.
21. Glasper E, McEwing G, Richardson J. Oxford handbook of children's and young people's nursing. 2011 (2nd ed.). New York: Oxford University Press.
22. Thomas Y, Price L. Drug use trajectories among minority youth. Dordrecht: Springer Netherlands. 1st ed. 2016, p. 38.
23. Leo MA, Lieber CS. Alcohol, vitamin A, and β-carotene: adverse interactions, including hepatotoxicity and carcinogenicity. Am J Clin Nutr 1999; 69(6):1071–1085. https://doi.org/10.1093/ajcn/69.6.1071
24. Mahdavinia M, Tobin MC, Fierstein JL, et al. African American Children Are More Likely to Be Allergic to Shellfish and Finfish: Findings from FORWARD, a Multisite Cohort Study. J Allergy Clin Immunol Pract 2021 Jul;9(7):2867-2873.e1. doi: 10.1016/j.jaip.2020.12.026.
25. Blaner WS. Vitamin A and provitamin A carotenoids. In: Marriott BP, Birt DF, Stallings VA, Yates AA, eds. Present Knowledge in Nutrition. 11th ed. Cambridge, Massachusetts: Wiley-Blackwell; 2020:73-91.).

CHAPTER TEN

UNDERSTANDING REDUCED RISKS OF DISEASE

People of West Central African descent are at reduced risk of severe morbidity and of mortality from malaria, dengue hemorrhagic fever (DHF) and yellow fever, tending to be asymptomatic or to display only mild or moderate symptoms compared to the typically more severe signs and symptoms shown by people of other ethnicities.[1-5]

DHF is the most significant mosquito-borne viral disease worldwide in terms of illness, mortality, and economic cost. Approximately 50-100 million new dengue virus infections occur annually of which up to 500,000 cases are hemorrhagic fever/dengue shock syndrome (DHF/DSS), the potentially most life-threatening form of the disease. The death rate from DHF/DSS is about 5%, mostly in children under age 15. The main features of DHF/DSS are severe arthralgia, bone pain, thrombocytopenia, increased vascular permeability, headache, gastrointestinal symptoms, and liver involvement.[6] Based on strong similarities between the features of DHF and those of vitamin A toxicity, the author proposed that DHF is an acute endogenous form of hypervitaminosis A.[7] The hypothesis is that dengue virus interacts with retinoids within the hepatic cell nuclei, causing retinoic acid receptor (RAR) activation and expression and cholestatic liver dysfunction. This impairs the mobilization and secretion of retinol-binding protein and lowers serum retinol concentrations but simultaneously results in the spillage of stored retinoids into the circulation in toxic concentrations, inducing the signs and symptoms of the disease. In one report, serum retinol was reduced in acute DHF,[8] as predicted, but retinyl ester and retinoic acid concentrations do not appear to have been measured in DHF and remain unknown.

Yellow fever is an acute viral hemorrhagic disease transmitted by infected mosquitoes of the Aedes aegypti species and is endemic in tropical areas of Africa and Central and South America.[9] In earlier centuries, yellow fever was transported to North America and Europe, causing major epidemics in the US. More than 41,000 deaths from yellow fever were reported in New Orleans from 1817-1905. The last major outbreak occurred in 1905, also in New Orleans, with the loss of 5,000 lives,

Like dengue, the yellow fever virus targets the liver and has many parallels to DHF.[10] Symptoms include fever, headache, muscle pain, thrombocytopenia, jaundice, nausea, vomiting and fatigue. A small proportion of patients develop severe symptoms that include bleeding from the mouth, nose, eyes, or stomach, leading to death within 7 to 10 days.

The contention that West Central Africans are less prone to die from yellow fever than Europeans has been challenged as racist and as having no analogous counterpart to the well-documented survival advantage associated with endemic exposure to Plasmodium falciparum infection.[11] Different degrees of severity of yellow fever are consistently observed across diverse populations. The first demonstration of a significant association between ancestry and the outcome of yellow fever was based on the analysis of data on European and African Americans during 19th century epidemics in the US. The analysis included incidence, mortality and case-fatality rates as well as socioeconomic, environmental, cultural, and demographic factors and acquired immunity status, which could have influenced the observed differences. There were no significant differences in incidence rates, but ancestral differences in mortality and case fatality rates were statistically significant for all epidemics tested ($P < 0.01$). European Americans with yellow fever were 6.8 times more likely to die than African Americans, and no other factor was significantly associated with mortality differences between the groups. It was concluded that the markedly lower yellow fever mortality rates for individuals of African ancestry were the result of human genetic variation in loci encoding innate immune mediators, and that discovery of characteristic host factors could prove valuable in the prevention of epidemics and the development of effective treatments.[12]

Plasmodium species parasites, yellow fever virus and dengue viruses similarly target the liver, the major storage site of vitamin A, but through different mechanisms. *Plasmodia spp*. emerging from the liver invade and reproduce in the red blood cells, causing vitamin A to be carried and dispersed via the circulation, with signs and symptoms recently reported to be associated with increased concentrations of retinoic acid.[13A] On the proposed theory, the yellow fever and dengue viruses directly result in liver damage, causing stored retinoids to be released into the circulation, thereby inducing the respective diseases.

It is suggested that West Central Africans and their descendants are protected from the lethal outcomes of these diseases due to the proposed evolutionary physiological adaptations: 1) sequestration of vitamin A away from the liver to subcutaneous adipose tissue and other organs, thus reducing its accessibility to the invading organisms; and 2) reduced vitamin A metabolism, causing it to accumulate to sub-toxic concentrations, thereby weakening the organisms and reducing the risk of severe disease.

Mechanism of Quinoline Drug Treatment for Malaria

Slowing the metabolism and secretion of vitamin A, causing it to accumulate to subtoxic levels and weaken the parasites, would likely involve the *dehydrogenase enzymes* that metabolize vitamin A. This could explain the mechanisms underlying the effectiveness of certain treatments for malaria; in particular, the 8-aminoquinoline class of drugs, including primaquine and tafenoquine, both of which target the liver-stage parasites.[13] Aldehyde dehydrogenase is selectively inhibited by quinolines. Other known inhibitors of ALDH1 are also lethal to or inhibit the growth of *P. falciparum* in vitro.[14] Since retinoic acid is produced from the oxidation of retinol to retinal via alcohol dehydrogenase, and from retinaldehyde via an aldehyde dehydrogenase reaction, the quinolines likely act as dehydrogenase inhibitors. These observations suggest that dehydrogenase inhibition – leading to the accumulation of vitamin A to concentrations sufficient to weaken *P. falciparum* – could represent a successful evolutionary adaptation to parasitic infection (see Chapter 12 – Reduced vitamin A metabolism and catabolism).

Understanding Reduced Disease Risk: The Case of NAFLD

African Americans have a lower percentage of liver fat and lower rates of NAFLD than European Americans[15,16] as well as more subcutaneous adipose tissue than Europeans or Hispanics. These findings may have resulted from the hypothesized adaptation involving the sequestration of vitamin A from the liver to other tissues. Vitamin A has a known role in liver damage.[17,18] For instance, retinoid metabolites extracted from rat liver tissues caused marked liver cell damage in a dose- and time-dependent manner, due to apoptosis.[19] Vitamin A can activate liver cells and potentiate liver damage in the absence of other hepatotoxins, such as alcohol.[20] The nonparenchymal Ito (or stellate) cells contain about 90% of total liver vitamin A and are the primary source of the extracellular matrix deposition involved in liver fibrosis.[21] During hepatic fibrosis these normally quiescent vitamin A-storing stellate cells transform into myofibroblastic cells and lose their intracellular droplets of retinyl esters.

The loss of retinyl esters increases retinoic acid and facilitates liver fibrogenesis.[22] Hence, the proposed adaptation of sequestering vitamin A away from the liver may not only have reduced the capacity of the malaria parasites to absorb vitamin A and use it to cause disease but could also have reduced the risk of African Americans developing NAFLD.

Dengue Hemorrhagic Fever and Yellow Fever – Switch from Mild to Severe Disease

The proposed adaptation of sequestering vitamin A from the liver to subcutaneous adipose tissue and other organs may explain the reduced risk of severe DHF and yellow fever to West Central Africans. Since these viral infections target the liver, the risk of severe illness may be lessened due to the presumably lower amounts of vitamin A in the damaged liver and hence lower quantity of stored vitamin A entering the circulation following infection. However, with increasing adoption of the typical US dairy-based diet, Africans and African Americans who develop fatty liver and associated features of the metabolic syndrome, including hypertension and diabetes, may be at increased risk of severe DHF due to slowed vitamin A metabolism and greater accumulation of and sensitivity to vitamin A. In fact, significant risk factors for DHF include diabetes mellitus, hypertension and obesity, all of which are associated with NAFLD.[23] In a matched case-control study in Brazil, individuals of African descent who reported being treated for hypertension were 13-fold more likely to acquire DHF than those not under treatment for hypertension.[24] Thus, with increasing NAFLD and associated liver dysfunction, African Americans would be at greater risk of DHF as well as diabetes and related diseases compared to European Americans, even with liver enzymes in the "normal" range.

References

1. Adu B, Dodoo D, Adukpo S, Gyan BA, Hedley PL, Goka B, et al. Polymorphisms in the RNASE3 Gene Are Associated with Susceptibility to Cerebral Malaria in Ghanaian Children. PLoS ONE 2011; 6(12): e29465. https://doi.org/10.1371/journal.pone.0029465
2. Halstead SB, Streit TG, Lafontant J, et al. Haiti: absence of dengue hemorrhagic fever despite hyperendemic dengue virus transmission. Am J Trop Med 2001; 65(3):180-183.
3. Sierra B, Kouri G, Guzman MG. Race: a risk factor for dengue hemorrhagic fever. Arch Virol 2007; 52:533-543.

4. McGuire RA, Coelho PRP. Parasites, Pathogens, and Progress: Diseases and Economic Development. Cambridge, MA: MIT Press, 2011.
5. Gainor EM, Harris E, LaBeaud AD. Uncovering the Burden of Dengue in Africa: Considerations on Magnitude, Misdiagnosis, and Ancestry. Viruses. 2022 Jan 25;14(2):233. doi: 10.3390/v14020233. PMID: 35215827; PMCID: PMC8877195.
6. Kalayanarooj S. Clinical Manifestations and Management of Dengue/DHF/DSS. Trop Med Health 2011; Dec;39(4 Suppl):83-7. doi: 10.2149/tmh.2011-S1088.
7. Mawson AR. Retinoids, race, and the pathogenesis of dengue hemorrhagic fever. Medical Hypotheses 2013; 81(6):1069–1074. doi: 10.1016/j.mehy.2013.08.004.
https://pubmed.ncbi.nlm.nih.gov/23999008/
8. Klassen P, Biesalski HK, Mazariegos M, Solomons NW, Fürst P. Classic dengue fever affects levels of circulating antioxidants. Nutrition 2004; 20(6):542-7.
9. WHO. Yellow fever.
https://www.who.int/news-room/fact-sheets/detail/yellow-fever
(Accessed October 4, 2022).
10. Quaresma JA, Barros VL, Pagliari C, Fernandes ER, Guedes F, Takakura CF, Andrade HF Jr, Vasconcelos PF, Duarte MI. Revisiting the liver in human yellow fever: virus-induced apoptosis in hepatocytes associated with TGF-beta, TNF-alpha and NK cells activity. Virology 2006; 345(1):22-30.
11. Espinosa M. The question of racial immunity to yellow fever in history and historiography. Social Science History 2014; 38(3–4):437–453. http://www.jstor.org/stable/90017043
12. Blake LE, Garcia-Blancoa MA. Human genetic variation and yellow fever mortality during 19th century U.S. epidemics. mBio 2014; 5(3). e01253-14 https://doi.org/10.1128/mBio.01253-14
13. Greenwood BM, Fidock DA, Kyle DE, Kappe SH, Alonso PL, Collins FH, Duffy PE. Malaria: progress, perils, and prospects for eradication. J Clin Invest 2008; 118(4):1266-76. doi: 10.1172/JCI33996.
14. Na J, Khan A, Kim JK, Wadood A, Choe YL, Walker DI, Jones DP, Lim CS, Park YH. Discovery of metabolic alterations in the serum of patients infected with Plasmodium spp. by high-resolution metabolomics. Metabolomics. 2019 Dec 23;16(1):9.
doi: 10.1007/s11306-019-1630-2. PMID: 31872321.
15. Graves PR, Kwiek JJ, Fadden P, Ray R, Hardeman K, Coley AM, Foley M, Haystead TA. Discovery of novel targets of quinoline drugs in the human purine binding proteome. Mol Pharmacol 2002; 62:1364-1372.

16. Parr CL, Magnus MC, Karlstad Ø et al. Vitamin A and D intake in pregnancy, infant supplementation, and asthma development: the Norwegian Mother and Child Cohort. Am J Clin Nutr 2018; 0:1-10, https://doi.org/10.1093/ajcn/nqy016
17. Guerrero R, Vega GL, Grundy SM et al. Ethnic differences in hepatic steatosis: An insulin resistance paradox? Hepatology 2009; 49:791–801. doi:10.1002/hep.22726.
18. Dongiovanni P, Anstee Q, Valenti L. Genetic predisposition in NAFLD and NASH: Impact on severity of liver disease and response to treatment. Curr Pharm Design 2013; 19(29), 5219–5238.
19. Cheruvattath, R., Orrego, M., Gautam, M., Byrne, T., Alam, S., Voltchenok, M., Edwin, M., Wilkens, J., Williams, J.W. and Vargas, H.E. (2006), Vitamin A toxicity: When one a day doesn't keep the doctor away. Liver Transpl, 12: 1888-1891. https://doi.org/10.1002/lt.21007
20. Saeed A, Dullaart RPF, Schreuder TCMA, Blokzijl H, Faber KN. Disturbed vitamin A metabolism in non-alcoholic fatty liver disease (NAFLD). Nutrients. 2017 Dec 29;10(1):29. doi: 10.3390/nu10010029.
21. Dan Z, Popov Y, Patsenker E, Preimel D, Liu C, Wang XD, et al. Hepatotoxicity of alcohol-induced polar retinol metabolites involves apoptosis via loss of mitochondrial membrane potential. FASEB J 2005; 19(7):845–7.
22. Sim W, Abril E, Earnest D. Mechanisms of Kupffer cell activation in hypervitaminosis A. In: Wisse E, Knook D, Decker K, editors. Cells of the hepatic sinusoid. Riiswijk: The Kupffer Cell Foundation; 1989, pp. 91–3.
23. Li D, Friedman SL. Liver fibrogenesis and the role of hepatic stellate cells: new insights and prospects for therapy. J Gastroenterol Hepatol 1999; 17: 618–33.
24. Tsuchida T, Friedman SL. Mechanisms of hepatic stellate cell activation. Nat Rev Gastroenterol Hepatol 2017; 14(7):397-411. doi: 10.1038/nrgastro.2017.38.
25. Deparis X, Maréchal V, Matheus S. Pathophysiological mechanisms of dengue fever: critical review of current concepts. Med Trop (Mars) 2009; 69(4):351–7.
26. Figueiredo MA, Rodrigues LC, Barreto ML, Lima JW, Costa MC, Morato V, et al. Allergies and diabetes as risk factors for dengue hemorrhagic fever: results of a case-control study. PLoS Negl Trop Dis 2010; 4(6):e699.

CHAPTER ELEVEN

THE COMPLICATIONS AND ADVERSE OUTCOMES OF PREGNANCY

The natural history, complications and adverse outcomes of pregnancy are not fully understood but their impact on society is immense. In 2019, the costs of maternal morbidity for all births in the US, from conception to age five, were estimated to reach $32.3 billion, combining the costs for treatment, hospitalization, social services and loss of economic productivity.[1] In approximate temporal order of occurrence during gestation, these risks include insulin resistance, elevated blood sugar (gestational diabetes), hypertension, proteinuria and edema (preeclampsia), seizures (eclampsia), third trimester hemolysis, elevated liver enzymes and low platelet count (HELLP syndrome), cardiovascular disease, birth before 37 weeks of pregnancy [preterm labor, the leading cause of infant mortality in the U.S.], birth defects, stillbirth, and postpartum depression. The most common contributors to maternal death in the first week postpartum are severe bleeding, high blood pressure, and infection, while cardiomyopathy is the leading cause of late deaths.[2]

Complications of pregnancy and adverse birth outcomes are 2-3 times more common in African American than in European American women[3] and have persisted for decades. African American women have over three times higher rates of pregnancy-related mortality than European American women (41.4 vs. 13.7 per 100,000), as well as higher rates of preterm birth, low birthweight births, and infant mortality. In a review of these facts, which were attributed to reduced socioeconomic advantage and to structural racism, the authors concluded: "Notably, disparities in maternal and infant health persist even when controlling for certain underlying social and economic factors, such as education and income, pointing to the roles racism and discrimination play in driving disparities".[4]

A Role for the Liver in Pregnancy, Its Complications and Adverse Outcomes

In seeking to understand the natural history, complications, and adverse outcomes of pregnancy in general, a role for the liver appears to be central. In the US population, the prevalence of nonalcoholic fatty liver disease (NAFLD) – defined as >5% of the liver's weight as fat – is estimated at >34%[5] and is associated with increased obesity, type 2 diabetes, and metabolic syndrome.[6]

Fatty liver in pregnancy occurs in two forms: chiefly as NAFLD, often linked to obesity, with a prevalence of about 10%, and rarely as acute fatty liver of pregnancy (AFLP), a serious condition that can lead to liver failure, occurring in about 0.5% of pregnancies.[7]

A central role for NAFLD in understanding the complications of pregnancy is shown by its association with increased risks of gestational diabetes, hypertensive complications and multiple adverse fetal outcomes.[8] In a study of temporal trends in NAFLD in pregnancies after 20 weeks gestation, based on discharge data on over 18 million pregnancies from the US national inpatient sample, pregnancies with NAFLD nearly tripled in recent years, from 10.5/100,000 pregnancies in 2007 to 28.9/100,000 in 2015. NAFLD during pregnancy was associated with gestational diabetes (23%), hypertensive complications (16%), postpartum hemorrhage (6%), preterm birth (9%), and possibly maternal death. The authors concluded that NAFLD should be considered a high-risk obstetric condition, with implications for pre-conception counseling and pregnancy care.[9]

What has been missing is a unifying theory connecting liver function with the natural history of pregnancy, its complications, and adverse outcomes. A common feature both of full term and preterm birth is rupture of the fetal membranes, in which retinoids play a major role.[10] Retinol declines in the serum during pregnancy but it increases in the liver,[11,12] activating the vitamin A-containing liver stellar cells as it progressively accumulates.[13] The resulting mild cholestasis, associated with the slowing of bile from liver into the duodenum, is followed by the increasing spillage of bile into the circulation.[14] Stored retinoids are also hypothesized to spill into the circulation in toxic concentrations, such that at nine months of gestation these compounds begin to destabilize and rupture the fetal membranes, leading to the onset of labor and parturition. On this hypothesis, disturbances in liver function occurring earlier in pregnancy exposing mother and fetus to excess retinoid concentrations could be the mechanism underling the pathogenesis of several forms of maternal morbidity as well as adverse birth and maternal outcomes. The appearance of specific conditions such as gestational diabetes and preeclampsia would thus depend on the concentration of circulating retinoids and on the timing of exposure.[15]

Gestational diabetes mellitus (GDM) and preeclampsia are both linked to fetal growth restriction (FGR) and to increased risks of later-onset vascular disease in mother and child.[16] The author and colleagues tested the retinoid toxicity hypothesis by determining retinoid concentration profiles in pregnant rats after the administration of the drug streptozotocin (STZ).[17, 18] STZ induced a GDM- and preeclampsia-like state that included elevated glucose levels and increased liver enzymes in the pregnant rats, followed by reduced pup weights, indicating fetal growth restriction (FGR). Blood pressure was slightly higher in the experimental group. As predicted, plasma retinol was significantly lower in the experimental dams than in the controls (0.45 vs. 1.04 μmol/L, $p = 0.0115$), as typically observed in gestational diabetes, preeclampsia, and preterm birth.[19]

The concentrations of retinyl esters and retinoic acid were also examined, apparently for the first time in an animal model of GDM and preeclampsia. The results are shown in the table below (Table 1-11). The percentage of retinyl esters, the ratio of retinyl esters to retinol, and the concentration of retinoic acid were all significantly higher than those of controls. The widely accepted standard of hypervitaminosis A in adults – percent retinyl esters >10% of total vitamin A (i.e., retinol plus esters)[20] was also exceeded (median 24% vs. 11% in the controls, $p = 0.008$), supporting the hypothesis that preeclampsia, gestational diabetes and FGR are causally linked to an endogenous form of retinoid toxicity associated with impaired liver function.

Table 1-11. Retinoid profiles in pregnant rats treated with streptozotocin (75 mg/kg) and controls.

	Control (n=10)	STZ (n=10)	p-value
Retinol (µmol/L) Median Range	1.04 0.38-1.37	0.45 0.16-0.68	0.0115
Total serum vitamin A (µmol/L) Median Range	1.24 0.53-2.01	0.78 0.58-2.10	0.2548
Total Ester (µmol/L) Median Range	0.13 0.03-0.49	0.22 0.09-1.75	0.1124
Ester/ROL Median Range	0.13 0.04-0.40	0.33 0.22-10.74	0.0045
% Ester Median Range	11.25 3.7-28.6	23.96 14.4-83.6	0.0082

	Control (n=8)	STZ (n=9)	p-value
All-trans RA (µmol/L) Median Range	0.0075 0.002-0.100	0.0155 0.0079-0.1065	0.0454

An important implication of these results is that retinol concentrations below the currently accepted cutoff for low serum retinol (<0.7 µmol/L)[21] do not necessarily indicate a state of vitamin A deficiency; they could instead be due to impaired hepatic mobilization and secretion. When considered in the context of additional measures of vitamin A (i.e., retinyl esters, the ratio of retinyl esters to total vitamin A, and retinoic acid), low serum retinol may in fact indicate the opposite state, i.e., the presence of vitamin A toxicity, as observed in the STZ study. Retinoid concentration profiling in pregnancy could therefore provide a more informative picture of vitamin A nutritional status and of pregnancy-related and birth outcomes than serum retinol alone.

It is not yet known to what extent these results apply to African Americans and women of other ancestral backgrounds. A report that pregnant African American women have a high rate of vitamin A "deficiency", based exclusively on low serum retinol levels,[22] calls for studies of retinoid concentration profiles in African Americans and other groups. Based on the foregoing, it is hypothesized that retinoid concentration profiling will show that while retinol levels are low in pregnancy in African Americans, percent retinyl esters and retinoic acid concentrations will be more consistent with a profile suggesting hypervitaminosis A.

Maternal Mortality: Genetic Risks

In the United States, African Americans are at significantly increased risk of maternal mortality than European Americans. A study of death certificate data from 2016 and 2017 showed that during pregnancy or within six weeks post-partum, African American women were five times more likely to die from cardiomyopathy and blood pressure disorders than European American women. They were also twice as likely to die from hemorrhage or embolism and six times as likely to die from cardiomyopathy between six weeks and one year postpartum.[23] In fact, over 90% of maternal deaths worldwide occur in sub-Saharan Africa and south Asia, mostly related to complications of pregnancy that include preeclampsia. An established determinant of preeclampsia is failure of placentation and of the physiological transformation of spiral arteries, leading to a poorly perfused placenta.[24] This underlying pathogenesis also relates to FGR, stillbirth, abruptio placentae, and preterm birth. A review of the literature concluded that indigenous African women and women of African ancestry are at greater risk of preeclampsia than other racial groups, and part of this susceptibility is due to genetic factors.[25]

A role for genetic factors in explaining these differences in maternal mortality is suggested by reports that allelic variants in the gene for apolipoprotein LI, APOL1, are found only in populations of African ancestry, and they contribute significantly to risks for chronic kidney disease and HIV-associated nephropathy (HIVAN), to which African Americans are also at increased risk.[26] Apolipoprotein L1 (APOL1), a gene located on chromosome 22, has two coding variants, G1 and G2, that are protective against parasitic diseases, notably *Trypanosoma brucei* infection (African sleeping sickness). Studies suggest that these APOL1 variants also contribute risk for preeclampsia. In a study of nearly 700 deliveries from African American women, associations between fetal APOL1 genotype and preeclampsia were evaluated using uncomplicated term pregnancies as controls. The infant APOL1 genotype was significantly associated with preeclampsia in a dominant inheritance pattern (Odds Ratio 1.41, p=0.029, 95% CI 1.037, 1.926), but not with pathological changes or other perinatal observations.[27]

Transgenic mice created to model the expression of intracellular APOL1 also developed preeclamptic or eclamptic seizures and had small litter sizes,[28] confirming the role of genetic factors in preeclampsia and indicating that infants carrying copies of APOL1 risk variants increase the risk of preeclampsia in African Americans [Note that APOL1G0 refers to APOL1 nonrisk allele vs. increased toxic functionality in G1/G2 variants]. These results suggest that screening for APOL1 may help to predict at-risk pregnancies, and targeted interventions could be developed to improve pregnancy outcomes; they also provide a further illustration of how protection against a tropical infectious disease may be associated with increased risks from other diseases.

The likely role of retinoid toxicity in preeclampsia likewise suggests a role for retinoids in the pathogenesis of APOL1 gene-associated disease. This is supported by a study of mice intraperitoneally injected with recombinant ApoL1 every other day for 3 months. The mice exhibited an enhanced dose-dependent expression of inflammation and apoptotic markers in kidney and serum compared to controls; these included the retinoic acid-induced gene protein I (RIG-I/NF-kB) signaling pathway. Conversely, knockdown of RIG-I significantly mitigated the ApoL1-induced upregulation of inflammatory and apoptotic markers in human podocytes, specialized cells that control the glomerular filtration apparatus.[29]

Given the importance of the liver in pregnancy-related conditions, what could explain the paradoxical observations that African American women are at increased risk of those conditions and of associated adverse outcomes despite having lower rates of NAFLD, NASH, and advanced fibrosis?[30] In a study of NAFLD in 700 pregnancies, 42.1 percent of the patients with NAFLD were White, 38.2 percent were Hispanic, and only 7.4 percent were Black.[31]

The postulated adaptations – namely, sequestering vitamin A away from the liver, and the tendency toward reduced vitamin A metabolism, hence increased overall vitamin A accumulation – could account for these facts. For instance, the increased risk and greater likelihood of death in African Americans from reproductive system diseases, including breast cancer, cervical cancer, and fibroids could reflect increased and potentially toxic concentrations of retinoids in the affected tissues. Earlier age of the onset of puberty in African American females could similarly reflect greater concentrations of retinoids in the reproductive system than in European American females.[32]

Even with lower levels of liver fat, African Americans may be more sensitive to vitamin A as a toxin and more likely to experience inflammatory changes in the liver and other organs, indicated by increased liver enzymes, as well as more prone to obesity, hypertension, and diabetes and to severe manifestations and secondary consequences of these conditions. In support of this hypothesis, a long-term prospective study of liver enzymes and diabetes risk found that high levels of gamma-glutamyl transferase (GGT) were most strongly associated with diabetes, even at levels within the normal range. However, adjusted incidence rates of diabetes by quartiles of liver enzymes were higher in African Americans, suggesting that abnormal GGT levels long antedate the diagnosis of diabetes, especially in African Americans.[33] A study comparing African American and European American patients with NAFLD reported a lower intrahepatic triglyceride content in the presence of NAFLD in African Americans (25.0% versus 51.9%), but the prevalence rate and severity of NASH did not differ between ethnicities.[34] A review of studies on NAFLD prevalence, severity, and prognosis in population-based cohorts reported that NAFLD prevalence was highest in Hispanics, intermediate in Whites, and lowest in Blacks; the risk of NASH (nonalcoholic steatohepatitis) was higher in Hispanics and lower in Blacks, but the proportion of patients with significant fibrosis did not significantly differ among racial or ethnic groups.[35]

In another study based on data from the Third National Health and Nutrition Examination Survey (NHANES III, a nationwide probability sample of 39,695 persons aged 2 months and older published in 2008), patients diagnosed with NAFLD had higher overall mortality and liver-related mortality rates than the general US population, and African Americans with NAFLD had significantly higher rates of all-cause mortality than European Americans.[36] A recent study reported that African American patients hospitalized with NAFLD were significantly more likely to die in hospital or suffer acute liver failure and had longer hospital stays than European American patients hospitalized with NAFLD.[37]

Preterm Birth

The hypothesized role of vitamin A toxicity in preterm birth proposed by the author[15] was recently tested and confirmed. Metabolites reflecting the biochemical dynamics in pregnancy and parturition were analyzed in pregnant women between 16- and 41-weeks gestational age using metabolomic methods (Ultra-High Performance Liquid Chromatography-Quadrupole Time-of-Flight Mass Spectrometry and Liquid Chromatography Mass Spectrometry, LC-MS/MS) to identify and validate the plasma metabolic signatures. Fifteen metabolites were significantly different between the preterm group and the term birth group. Metabolic pathways involving retinol, linoleic acid, d-arginine, and d-ornithine were associated with preterm birth. Verification by LC-MS/MS, focusing on retinol metabolism, disclosed that retinol levels were significantly reduced in preterm birth compared to term birth, while retinal palmitate, all-trans-retinal, and 13-cis-retinoic acid (13cis-RA) significantly increased ($p < 0.05$). All-trans-retinal and 13cis-RA showed improved predictions for preterm birth-related retinol metabolites, suggesting that retinoid metabolism improves the accuracy of prediction for preterm birth.[38] This new finding suggests an additional outcome of altered retinoid metabolism in the complications of pregnancy, and for the use of a retinoid diagnostic biomarker.

In conclusion, this review supports the hypothesis that pregnancy and parturition are associated with sub-clinical hypervitaminosis A, and that the complications of pregnancy and of adverse birth and maternal outcomes may be related to an endogenous overall state of retinoid toxicity due to NAFLD and exposure of mother and fetus to hazardous concentrations of retinoids.[15] Pregnancy is already known as a state of insulin resistance.[39]

Due to the suggested evolutionary adaptations, people of West Central African descent may already be in a state of subclinical hypervitaminosis A. Studies are now needed to determine retinoid concentration profiles in pregnancy and its related complications and adverse birth and maternal outcomes in women of different ancestral backgrounds. An important implication of the thesis, further explored in the Appendices, is that reduced exposure to vitamin A through dietary restriction of dairy products and the adoption of traditional or modified West Central African diets could have an ameliorative impact on pregnancy-related complication and adverse outcomes.

References

1. So O'Neil et al., The High Costs of Maternal Morbidity Show Why We Need Greater Investment in Maternal Health (Commonwealth Fund, Nov. 2021). https://doi.org/10.26099/nz8s-4708
2. The Commonwealth Fund. Maternal Mortality and Maternity Care in the United States Compared to 10 Other Developed Countries. Issue Brief November 18, 2020. https://www.commonwealthfund.org/publications/issue-briefs/2020/nov/maternal-mortality-maternity-care-us-compared-10-countries (Accessed November 23, 2022).
3. Petersen EE, Davis NL, Goodman D, et al. Racial/Ethnic Disparities in Pregnancy-Related Deaths — United States, 2007–2016. MMWR Morb Mortal Wkly Rep 2019; 68:762–765. DOI: http://dx.doi.org/10.15585/mmwr.mm6835a3external
4. Hill L, Artiga S, Ranji U. Racial Disparities in Maternal and Infant Health: Current Status and Efforts to Address. Published: November 01, 2022. https://www.kff.org/racial-equity-and-health-policy/issue-brief/racial-disparities-in-maternal-and-infant-health-current-status-and-efforts-to-address-them/ (Accessed November 11, 2022.)
5. Kim D, Kim WR, Kim HJ, Therneau TM. Association between noninvasive fibrosis markers and mortality among adults with nonalcoholic fatty liver disease in the United States. Hepatology 2013; 57: 1357– 65.
6. Nureddin M, Ntanios F, Malhotra D, Hoover K, Emir B, McLeod E, et al. Predicting NAFLD prevalence in the United States using National Health and Nutrition Examination Survey 2017–2018 transient elastography data and application of machine learning. Hepatol Commun 2022; 6:1537– 1548. https://doi.org/10.1002/hep4.1935).
7. Azzaroli F, Mazzella G, Marchesini G et al. Fatty liver in pregnancy: a narrative review of two distinct conditions, Expert Review of Gastroenterology & Hepatology 2020; 14:2, 127-135, DOI: 10.1080/17474124.2020.1715210.
8. El Jamaly H, Eslick GD, Weltman M. Systematic review with meta-analysis: Non-alcoholic fatty liver disease and the association with pregnancy outcomes. Clin Mol Hepatol. 2022 Jan;28(1):52-66. doi: 10.3350/cmh.2021.0205.

9. Sarkar M, Grab J, Dodge JL, Gunderson EP et al. Non-alcoholic fatty liver disease in pregnancy is associated with adverse maternal and perinatal outcomes. J Hepatol. 2020 Sep;73(3):516-522. doi: 10.1016/j.jhep.2020.03.049.
10. Blanchon L, Marceau G, Borel V, Prat C et al. Étude de la voie des rétinoïdes au sein des membranes fœtales humaines: mise en évidence de gènes cibles [Implications of retinoid pathway in human fetal membranes: study of target genes]. Gynecol Obstet Fertil. 2011 Jun;39(6):370-2. French. doi: 10.1016/j.gyobfe.2011.04.009.
11. Bates CJ, Vitamin A in pregnancy and lactation. Proc Nutr Soc 1983; 42: 65-79.
12. Satre MA, Ugen KE, Kochhar DM. Developmental changes in endogenous retinoids during pregnancy and embryogenesis in the mouse. Biol Reprod 1992; 46: 802-810.
13. Peverill W, Powell LW, Skoien R. Evolving concepts in the pathogenesis of NASH: beyond steatosis and inflammation. Int J Mol Sci 2014; 15(5):8591–8638).
14. Wagner M, Trauner M. Recent advances in understanding and managing cholestasis. F1000 Research 2016 Apr 19; 5:F1000 Faculty Rev-705. doi: 10.12688/f1000research.8012.1.
15. Mawson AR. A role for the liver in parturition and preterm birth. J Transl Sci 2016; 2(3):154-159. doi: 10.15761/JTS.1000133. Epub 2016 Apr 18. PMID: 27595011; PMCID: PMC5010230.
16. Wu P. Obstetric outcomes and later cardiovascular risk. Gynecological Endocrinology 2021; 37:3:193-194, DOI: 10.1080/09513590.2021.1887119.
17. Mawson AR, Bennett W, Tanumihardjo S, Mills J, Smith A, Kirui P, May W, Martin JN Jr. Altered retinoid profiles in an animal model of preeclampsia, gestational diabetes, and fetal growth restriction. Presented at the 57th Annual Meeting of the Society for Gynecological Investigation, Orlando, FL. March 26, 2010; Reproductive Science 2010 Abstract 592. Vol. 17, Supplement.
18. Mawson AR. Method for diagnosing gestational diabetes, preeclampsia, and fetal growth restriction. United States Patent No. US 8,883,512 B1. Date of Patent: Nov. 11, 2014. https://patents.google.com/patent/US8883512B1/en
19. Radhika M, Bhaskaram P, Balakrishna N et al. Effects of vitamin A deficiency during pregnancy on maternal and child health. BJOG: An International Journal of Obstetrics & Gynaecology 2002; 109: 689-693. https://doi.org/10.1111/j.1471-0528.2002.01010.x

20. Krasinski SD, Russell RM, Otradovec CL, Sadowski JA et al. Relationship of vitamin A and vitamin E intake to fasting plasma retinol, retinol-binding protein, retinyl esters, carotene, alpha-tocopherol, and cholesterol among elderly people and young adults: increased plasma retinyl esters among vitamin A-supplement users. Am J Clin Nutr. 1989 Jan;49(1):112-20. doi: 10.1093/ajcn/49.1.112. PMID: 2911996.
21. Tanumihardjo SA, Russell RM, Stephensen CB, Gannon BM, Craft NE et al. Biomarkers of Nutrition for Development (BOND)—Vitamin A Review. The Journal of Nutrition 2016; 146(9):1816S–1848S. https://doi.org/10.3945/jn.115.229708
22. Suzuki M, Wang T, Garretto D, Isasi CR, Cardoso WV, Greally JM, Quadro L. Disproportionate vitamin A deficiency in women of specific ethnicities linked to differences in allele frequencies of vitamin A-related polymorphisms. Nutrients 2021 May 21;13(6):1743. doi: 10.3390/nu13061743. PMID: 34063790; PMCID: PMC8223783.
23. MacDorman MF et al. Racial and ethnic disparities in maternal mortality in the United States using enhanced vital records, 2016–2017. American Journal of Public Health 2021; 111(9):1673-81.
24. Redman CWG, Sargent IL. Immunological factors and placentation: implications for pre-eclampsia. In: Lyall F, Belfort M, eds. Pre-eclampsia. Cambridge (United Kingdom): Cambridge University Press; 2007.
25. Nakimuli A, Chazara O, Byamugisha J, Elliott AM et al. Pregnancy, parturition and preeclampsia in women of African ancestry. Am J Obstet Gynecol. 2014 Jun;210(6):510-520.e1. doi: 10.1016/j.ajog.2013.10.879. Epub 2013 Oct 30. PMID: 24184340; PMCID: PMC4046649.
26. Goyal R, Singhal PC. APOL1 risk variants and the development of HIV-associated nephropathy. FEBS J. 2021 Oct;288(19):5586-5597. doi: 10.1111/febs.15677. Epub 2020 Dec 31. PMID: 33340240; PMCID: PMC8213861.
27. Miller AK, Azhibekov T, O'Toole JF, Sedor JR et al. Association of preeclampsia with infant APOL1 genotype in African Americans. BMC Med Genet 2020; 21, 110. https://doi.org/10.1186/s12881-020-01048-4
28. Bruggeman LA, Wu Z, Luo L et al. APOL1-G0 protects podocytes in a mouse model of HIV-associated nephropathy. PLoS One 2019 Oct 29; 14(10):e0224408. doi: 10.1371/journal.pone.0224408. PMID: 31661509; PMCID: PMC6818796.
29. Fang J, Yao X, Hou M, Duan M, Xing L, Huang J, Wang Y, Zhu B, Chen Q, Wang H. ApoL1 induces kidney inflammation through RIG-I/NF-κB activation. Biochem Biophys Res Commun. 2020 Jun

25;527(2):466-473. doi: 10.1016/j.bbrc.2020.04.054. Epub 2020 Apr 24. PMID: 32336543.
30. Browning MG, Khoraki J, DeAntonio JH, et al. Protective effect of black relative to white race against non-alcoholic fatty liver disease in patients with severe obesity, independent of type 2 diabetes. Int J Obes (Lond) 2018; 42: 926- 929.
31. Sarkar M, Grab J, Dodge JL, Gunderson EP et al. Non-alcoholic fatty liver disease in pregnancy is associated with adverse maternal and perinatal outcomes. J Hepatol 2020 Sep;73(3):516-522. doi: 10.1016/j.jhep.2020.03.049.
32. Owen CM, Goldstein EH, Clayton JA, Segars JH. Racial and ethnic health disparities in reproductive medicine: an evidence-based overview. Semin Reprod Med 2013 Sep;31(5):317-24. doi: 10.1055/s-0033-1348889.
33. Schneider AL, Lazo M, Ndumele CE et al. Liver enzymes, race, gender and diabetes risk: the Atherosclerosis Risk in Communities (ARIC) Study. Diabet Med 2013; 30(8):926-33. doi: 10.1111/dme.12187.
34. Bril F, Cusi K. Response to comment on Bril et al. Clinical and histologic characterization of nonalcoholic steatohepatitis in African American patients. Diabetes Care 2018;41:187-192. Diabetes Care 2018; 41: e137- e138.
35. Rich NE, Oji S, Mufti AR, Browning JD, Parikh ND et al. Racial and ethnic disparities in nonalcoholic fatty liver disease prevalence, severity, and outcomes in the United States: A Systematic Review and Meta-analysis. Clin Gastroenterol Hepatol. 2018 Feb;16(2):198-210.e2. doi: 10.1016/j.cgh.2017.09.041.
36. Younossi ZM, Otgonsuren M, Venkatesan C et al. In patients with non-alcoholic fatty liver disease, metabolically abnormal individuals are at a higher risk for mortality while metabolically normal individuals are not. Metabolism 2013; 62:352-360.
37. Lee DU. The racial disparity in hospital outcomes of African-American and white patients with nonalcoholic fatty liver disease: analysis of 2011-2017 US hospitals DDW ePoster Library. Lee D. 05/22/21; 320149; Sa346.
https://eposters.ddw.org/ddw/2021/ddw-2021-virtual/320149/david.lee.the.racial.disparity.in.hospital.outcomes.of.african-american.and.html?f=menu%3D14%2Abrowseby%3D8%2Asortby%3D2%2Amedia%3D3%2Aspeaker%3D851571 (Accessed November 16, 2022). NAFLD outcomes worse for Blacks. Gastroenterology & Endoscopy News August 11, 2021

https://www.gastroendonews.com/In-the-News/Article/08-21/NAFLD-Outcomes-Worse-for-Blacks/64226 (Accessed November 16, 2022).

38. You YA, Hwang SY, Kim SM et al. Identification of Indicators for Preterm Birth Using Retinoid Metabolites. Metabolites 2021 Jul 7;11(7):443. doi: 10.3390/metabo11070443. PMID: 34357337; PMCID: PMC830476.
39. CDC. Gestational diabetes. August 10, 2021. https://www.cdc.gov/diabetes/basics/gestational.html#:~:text=During%20pregnancy%2C%20your%20body%20makes,your%20body's%20need%20for%20insulin

CHAPTER TWELVE

REDUCED VITAMIN A METABOLISM AND CATABOLISM

Observing that red blood cell disorders such as sickle cell anemia and the thalassemias were highly prevalent in tropical areas where malaria was endemic, the geneticist J.B.S. Haldane hypothesized that the disorders were common in these regions because natural selection had created biological traits that are protective against lethal or severe malaria.[1] Haldane's hypothesis was confirmed by A. C. Allison, who showed that the geographical distribution of the sickle-cell mutation in the beta hemoglobin gene (HBB) was limited to Africa and correlated with malaria endemicity, and individuals who carried the sickle cell trait – possessing the sickle cell gene from one rather than both parents – were resistant to malaria.[2] A striking worldwide geographical difference also exists for a mutation in the Duffy antigen gene (FY), which encodes a membrane protein used by the *Plasmodium vivax* malaria parasite to enter red blood cells. This mutation disrupts the protein, conferring protection against *P. vivax* malaria, and is pervasive throughout sub-Saharan Africa but is rare outside of Africa.[3]

The origin of these traits and understanding the manifestations of the disorders have remained uncertain, but they can be tentatively explained by the second hypothesized evolutionary adaptation to endemic parasitism proposed here: that reduced or slowed vitamin A metabolism and catabolism cause it to accumulate to sub-toxic concentrations and weaken the parasites, thereby reducing the risk of severe disease. Over an evolutionary timescale, these suggested mutations in the metabolism of vitamin A could also account for the unique health profile of people of West Central African descent, and for their susceptibility to many chronic diseases common in North America. This profile includes sickle cell anemia (SCA) and glucose-6-phosphate dehydrogenase deficiency (G6PDd).

Both sickle cell trait and G6PDd are protective against death from cerebral malaria. SCA occurs in about 1 in 500 live births and affects 90,000 to 100,000 people in the US, mainly African Americans. Alteration of a single nucleotide in the gene for the beta chain of the hemoglobin protein, hemoglobin S (HbS), results in rigid, sickle-shaped red blood cells that typically appear around 6 months of age. SCA is associated with attacks of severe pain, swelling of the extremities, bacterial infections, and increased risks of kidney disease, retinopathy and stroke.[4] Sickle cell trait affects 1-3 million Americans, 8-10% of African Americans, and >100 million people worldwide. Unlike sickle cell disease, where two genes, one from each parent, cause the production of abnormal hemoglobin, individuals with sickle cell trait carry only one defective gene and typically have few or no medical problems.[5]

G6PDd is an X-linked recessive inborn error of metabolism that predisposes to hemolysis in response to stress and the consumption of certain foods, notably fava beans. Symptoms such as jaundice, dark urine, shortness of breath, and fatigue may develop, but most people with the condition are asymptomatic and many never have symptoms. G6PDd is the most common human congenital defect of metabolism, defined by decreased NADPH+H(+) and a reduced form of glutathione. It is associated with susceptibility to Alzheimer's disease[6] and contributes to the pathophysiology of cerebral vasculopathy in children with SCA.[7] Among African American neonates, a subgroup of G6PDd infants have elevated rates of hemolysis, a higher incidence of hyperbilirubinemia, and a greater requirement for phototherapy compared with G6PD-normal neonate controls.[8]

Recalling that the retinoid-converting enzymes include retinol dehydrogenase, alcohol dehydrogenase, aldo-keto reductase, and aldehyde dehydrogenase,9 [171] the mechanism underlying the health profile of people of West Central African descent may involve an overall reduction of dehydrogenase enzyme activity such that, in the dairy-based dietary environment of North America, it could lead to an accumulation of vitamin A and the noted adverse health outcomes. The incidence of osteoporosis and related fractures in African American women is half that of European American women, but an exponential increase in hip fracture rates occur in African American women over age 70, with those sustaining osteoporosis-related fractures experiencing increased disability and decreased survival.[10]

Consistent with the hypothesis of lower dehydrogenase enzyme activity, mice deficient in retinaldehyde dehydrogenase (which converts retinaldehyde to retinoic acid) have a higher trabecular and cortical bone mass compared to age- and sex-matched control mice; they also have increased cortical bone thickness, higher bone marrow adiposity, higher levels of bone morphogenetic protein, and enhanced osteoblastogenesis. Retinaldehyde accumulates in retinaldehyde dehydrogenase-deficient mice, and in vitro it strongly induces bone morphogenetic protein 2 (BMP2).[11]

Given that vitamin A intake is a known risk factor for osteoporosis and fractures,[12] these findings in mice deficient in retinaldehyde dehydrogenase suggest that in a largely parasite-free and vitamin A-rich dietary environment, lower retinaldehyde dehydrogenase enzyme activity could lead to an accumulation of vitamin A and to increased risks of osteoporosis, fractures, and other vitamin A toxicity-associated diseases. This could explain the fact that older African American women, despite having higher bone mineral densities (BMD) than European American women throughout life, are at significant risk of developing osteoporosis and of having poorer outcomes following diagnosis.

In patients with colorectal cancer, research on drug metabolism supports the hypothesis that lower dehydrogenase enzyme activity leads to an accumulation of vitamin A to toxic concentrations in the intestines. Dihydropyrimidine dehydrogenase (DPD) is the initial and rate-limiting enzyme of 5-fluorouracil (5-FU). Studies have linked reduced DPD activity to the development of 5-FU toxicity (i.e., leukopenia and anemia). African Americans with colorectal cancer have increased 5-FU–associated toxicity and decreased overall survival compared to European American patients. DPD enzyme activity in healthy African American volunteers was reported to be significantly reduced compared to that of healthy European American volunteers, with threefold higher rates of DPD deficiency in African Americans compared to European Americans (8.0% vs. 2.8%, respectively; $P = 0.07$).[13]

References

1. Haldane JBS. Diseases and evolution. Ricerca Science Supplement 1949; 19:3-10.
2. Allison AC. Protection afforded by sickle-cell trait against subtertian malarial infection. British Medical Journal 1954; 4857: 290–294.
3. Sabeti P. Natural selection: uncovering mechanisms of evolutionary adaptation to infectious disease. Nature Education 208; 1(1):13.
4. NHLBI. Sickle cell disease. https://www.nhlbi.nih.gov/health-topics/sickle-celldisease/health-professional-information (Accessed October 31, 2020).
5. American Society of Hematology, 2018. American Society of Hematology, 2018. http://www.hematology.org/Patients/Anemia/Sickle-Cell-Trait.aspx (Accessed October 31, 2020).

6. Evlice A, Ulusu NN. Glucose-6-phosphate dehydrogenase: a novel hope on a bloodbased diagnosis of Alzheimer's disease. Acta Neurol Belg 2017; 117(1):229-234. doi: 10.1007/s13760-016-0666-6.
7. 150. Joly P, Garnier N, Kebaili K et al. G6PD deficiency and absence of α-thalassemia increase the risk for cerebral vasculopathy in children with sickle cell anemia. Eur J Haematol 2016; 96(4):404-8. doi: 10.1111/ejh.12607.
8. Kaplan M, Herschel M, Hammerman C, Hoyer JD, Stevenson DK. Hyperbilirubinemia among African American, glucose-6-phosphate dehydrogenase-deficient neonates. Pediatrics. 2004 Aug;114(2):e213-9. doi: 10.1542/peds.114.2.e213. PMID: 15286259.
9. Hong SH, Kim KR, Oh DK. Biochemical properties of retinoid-converting enzymes and biotechnological production of retinoids. Appl Microbiol Biotechnol 2015; 99(19):7813-26. doi: 10.1007/s00253-015-6830-8.
10. Bohannon AD. Osteoporosis and African American women. J Women's Health & Gender-Based Medicine 1999; 8:609–15.
11. Nallamshetty S, Wang H, Rhee EJ et al. Deficiency of retinaldehyde dehydrogenase 1 induces BMP2 and increases bone mass in vivo. PLoS One 2013; 8(8):e71307. doi:10.1371/journal.pone.0071307.
12. Melhus H, Michaelsson K, Kindmark A et al. Excessive dietary intake of vitamin A Is associated with reduced bone mineral density and increased risk for hip fracture. Ann Intern Med 1998; 129:770–778. doi: 10.7326/0003-4819-129-10-199811150-00003
13. Mattison LK, Fourie J, Desmond RA et al. Increased prevalence of dihydropyrimidine dehydrogenase deficiency in African-Americans compared with Caucasians. Clin Cancer Res 2006; 12(18):5491-5495; DOI: 10.1158/1078-0432.CCR-06-074

CHAPTER THIRTEEN

SPECTRUM OF DEHYDROGENASE ENZYME ACTIVITY

Reduced metabolism vitamin A via dehydrogenase enzyme activity (and reduced clearance of retinoic acid by CYP26 enzymes) has been proposed as the second of two hypothesized evolutionary physiological adaptations to the threat of malaria infection; that is, causing vitamin A to accumulate to subtoxic concentrations and weaken the parasites, thereby reducing the risk of severe disease. Here we focus on vitamin A metabolism and postulate a spectrum of dehydrogenase enzyme activity in human populations.

It is hypothesized that reduced enzyme activity leads to increased vitamin A accumulation and to reduced risks of severe malaria but also to increased risks of vitamin A-associated chronic diseases. This scenario applies mainly to people of West Central Africa, probably to tropical areas in Southeast Asia that are exposed to endemic parasitism,[1] and to human populations exposed to vegetable-based dietary environments that are low in preformed vitamin A.[2] Conversely, higher enzyme activity is related to dairy-based dietary environments and reduced exposure to endemic parasitism.

Increased dehydrogenase enzyme activity and increased catabolism of vitamin A may be an ancestral adaptation to dependence on grazing animals,[3] including consumption of their milk and organ meats, which are rich in preformed vitamin A. This scenario is hypothesized to apply to people of northern European origin and to populations dependent on cows, sheep, and other grazing animals, including the Maasai people of Kenya and northern Tanzania. As noted, the traditional Maasai diet of milk, blood and meat, although rich in lactose, fat, cholesterol, and vitamin A, is associated with low blood cholesterol levels, low rates of cholelithiasis (especially cholesterol gallstones), low blood pressure, and low rates of atherosclerotic coronary artery disease.[4, 5] A genome-wide scan of HapMap 3 SNP data, aimed at identifying genomic regions under selection in the Maasai, identified regions containing genes involved in lactose and lipid metabolism, harboring genetic polymorphisms responsible for the unusual lipid metabolism and protection against heart diseases and lactose intolerance.[6] [HapMap 3 is the third phase of the International HapMap project. This phase increases the number of DNA samples covered, from 270 in phases I and II to 1,301 samples from a variety of human populations. See https://www.sanger.ac.uk/resources/downloads/human/hapmap3.html. Increased dehydrogenase enzyme activity, associated with rapid vitamin A metabolism and catabolism, could play an important role in lactase persistence and in protection against heart disease in the Maasai.

People of northern European descent are hypothesized to have an intermediate level of dehydrogenase enzyme activity and vitamin A catabolism, and of lactose persistence, arising from their historic dependence on grazing animals (see Figure 1-13). Pastoralism arose in Europe and East Africa 4,000–10,000 years ago,[7] leading to selection for lactase persistence. In a similar timespan to that in which lactase persistence was conferred in Europeans, selection pressure from their diet of milk, blood and meat may have resulted in genetic adaptations in the Maasai that protected them from atherosclerosis and heart disease.[8]

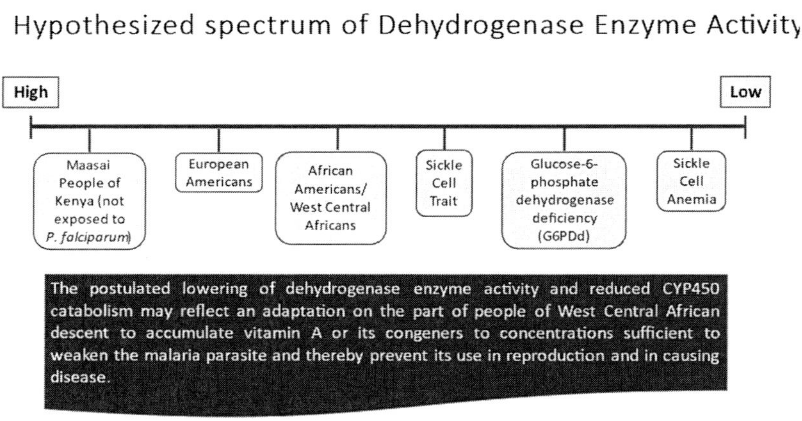

Figure 1-13. Hypothesized spectrum of dehydrogenase enzyme activity.

Further to the right on Figure 1-13, it is hypothesized that reduced dehydrogenase and/or CYP450 enzymatic catabolism of vitamin A in people of West Central African descent have resulted in its accumulation to subtoxic levels; that is, lower serum levels of retinol but higher concentrations of retinyl esters and retinoic acid, and higher ratios of retinyl esters to retinol. In the ancestral environment these features would serve to weaken *Plasmodia spp* and their ability to invade and reproduce in the red blood cells, thereby reducing the risk of severe malaria and representing a successful adaptation to endemic malaria parasitism. This hypothesized retinoid concentration profile, with increased circulating concentrations of retinyl esters and retinoic acid, could represent an inherited form of "vaccination" against severe malaria.

Individuals with sickle cell trait are notably at reduced risk of severe malaria and are hypothetically positioned on the spectrum to the right of people of West Central Africa as a group. They experience few symptoms except under extreme atmospheric conditions or dehydration when some of the same symptoms develop as in sickle cell anemia itself. Individuals with G6PD deficiency are likewise protected against severe malaria but can become severely anemic after consuming fava beans or when under stress. Here they are placed further to the right, towards the low end of the spectrum of dehydrogenase enzyme activity.

Sickle cell disease (sickle cell anemia, SCA) is hereditary hemolytic anemia. SCA is associated with low retinol levels.[9] However, SCA is also associated with severe chest and bone pain crises, which are often triggered by malaria.[10] The observation that malaria infection is associated with low concentrations of retinol but increased retinoic acid,[11] suggests that SCA may be similarly associated with retinoic acid.

The point mutation in the hemoglobin gene (HbS) that causes sickling is likewise hypothesized to have arisen from evolutionary physiological adaptations to endemic parasitism and, in the case of SCA, from mutations that entailed greater slowing or reductions in the catabolism of vitamin A. On this hypothesis, SCA represents an endogenous form or expression of retinoid toxicity. Subject to testing, the hypothesis suggests new avenues for the prevention and treatment of SCA-associated morbidity.

The conjecture that SCA is associated with retinoic acid is supported by the presence of Heinz bodies, which are intracellular precipitates of denatured hemoglobin found in abundance in the red blood cells of patients with sickle hemoglobinopathy.[12] Heinz bodies are the most visible expression of massive hemoglobin denaturation but in G6PD-deficient individuals they are seen in the erythrocytes only during hemolytic episodes.[13] In the thalassemias, G6PDd, and particularly in SCA, the oxidative degradation of hemoglobin S leads to hemichrome formation and precipitation as Heinz bodies. This is associated with shortened erythrocyte survival[14] and is proposed to result from reduced catabolism and increased accumulation of retinoic acid.

This hypothesis is supported by a study of the formation of Heinz bodies in kittens exposed to various diets. It was found that Heinz bodies could be induced using a commercial salmon-based diet containing 16.5 mg of nitrite, 39 mg of histamine, and 210,000 IU of vitamin A/kg of diet (dry-matter basis).[15] This study suggests that exposure to other high vitamin A diets, coupled with vitamin A accumulation due to reduced dehydrogenase enzyme activity, could cause hypervitaminosis A-induced anemia and the formation of Heinz bodies. Consistent with the hypothesis that CYP26 enzymatic activity is strongly reduced in SCA, leading to the accumulation of retinoic acid, hence chronic hypervitaminosis A and to the features of SCA, a study of CYP26 knockout mice compared to controls showed increased bone marrow cellularity and decreased frequency of erythroid progenitor cells in the bone marrow, i.e., hallmarks of SCA.[16] In addition, the CYP26a1 knockout decreased the clearance of exogenous all-trans-retinoic acid by 70% and increased its half-life sixfold.[17]

In long-term residents of sub-Saharan Africa, the hypothesized reduction in vitamin A enzyme activity may serve to protect against severe disease from malaria via vitamin A accumulation to sub-toxic levels, thereby weakening the parasite. However, in the environment of North America, lacking major vitamin A-absorbing parasitic organisms, the mainly dairy-based diet may increase risks of metabolic, malignant, and allergic disease. This may occur irrespective of ancestral origin or ethnicity, via the mechanisms of apoptosis, mitochondrial dysfunction, hyperuricemia, and increased ferritinemia,[18] especially in people of West Central African descent. Tendencies towards reduced vitamin A metabolism and catabolism, coupled with a high dietary intake and the absence of endemic parasitism, may create especially high risks of vitamin A-associated chronic inflammatory diseases.

The Causes of Hemolytic Anemia Revisited

Anemia is a common condition in which the number of red blood cells is lower than normal and the capacity of the blood to carry oxygen to the tissues is decreased. The primary indicator is hemoglobin (Hb) concentration: 14-17.5 grams per deciliter for men, and 12.3-15.3 gm/dL for women. The associated symptoms are fatigue, weakness, dizziness and shortness of breath. Of greater concern are increased risks of maternal and child mortality. The common causes of anemia are said to include nutritional deficiencies, including vitamin A, but particularly iron deficiency, hemoglobinopathies, and infectious diseases such as malaria, tuberculosis, HIV, and parasitic infections. It is estimated that 42% of children under age 5 years and 40% of pregnant women worldwide are anemic.[19] The prevalence of anemia among women of childbearing age in all West and Central African countries in 2010 was estimated to be above 50% among pregnant women and 40% among non-pregnant women.[20]

Anemia is 3.3-fold more common in African Americans than European Americans, and it is linked to vascular disease, hypertension, and diabetes.[21,22]

The main cause of anemia in preschool children worldwide is said to be iron deficiency, with vitamin A deficiency as a contributing factor.[23] Both iron and vitamin A are stored mainly in the liver, and inorganic iron is needed for hemoglobin synthesis.[24] Low iron intake and/or bioavailability are believed to be responsible for most anemia in industrialized countries and for about half of the anemia cases in developing countries; the other half is believed to be due mainly to malaria and blood loss from parasitic infections and other nutrient deficiencies.[25]

Vitamin A is importantly involved in the regulation of iron release from the liver, and iron deficiency is due to liver dysfunction and impaired mobilization and secretion of both iron and retinol.[26] Iron supplementation or repletion stimulates the release of iron and vitamin A by removing the inhibitory effect of iron deficiency on hepatic mobilization, and improves vitamin A metabolism after a previous state of iron deficiency.[27] Oral iron supplementation with ferrous sulfate (FeSO4) is therefore recommended to treat iron deficiency and prevent iron deficiency anemia.[28]

An alternative mechanism can be considered. Rather than a deficiency of iron or vitamin A, the joint occurrence of low serum iron and retinol could be due to their accumulation and impaired mobilization and secretion from the liver. Although iron supplementation can normalize both serum iron and retinol levels, hemolytic anemia may not be caused by iron deficiency; it could be secondary to vitamin A accumulation and impaired secretion, and a toxic effect due to liver dysfunction and the entry into the circulation of stored retinyl esters and/or retinoic acid, causing red blood cell damage.

Vitamin A toxicity is conjectured to be the primary cause of hemolytic anemia in acute infectious states such as malaria. Anemia is the primary clinical manifestation of severe malaria in children,[29] and acute malaria infection is associated with significantly increased serum concentrations of retinoic acid.[11] A contributory role for liver disease in the etiology of anemia is suggested by the fact that hemolytic anemia occurs in about 75% of patients with advanced liver disease.[30]

Anemia shares many signs in common with hypervitaminosis A: fatigue, weakness, pale or yellowish skin, irregular heartbeats, shortness of breath, dizziness or lightheadedness, cold extremities, headache, chest and bone pain.[31] Studies indicate that vitamin A interacts directly with cell membranes to increase their permeability and fluidity, causing hemolysis.[32,33]

Anemia is extremely common among hemodialysis patients and contributes to the signs and symptoms of reduced kidney function, including fatigue, depression, dyspnea and with increased morbidity and mortality related to cardiovascular disease.[34] In a study of patients with end-stage renal failure maintained on regular dialysis treatment, plasma vitamin A levels were inversely correlated with hematocrit, suggesting that raised plasma vitamin A levels in regular dialysis patients contribute to risks of anemia.[35]

Further support for the vitamin A toxicity hypothesis comes from an animal study aimed at determining whether iron deficiency alters the concentration of vitamin A in plasma or liver and the chemical distribution between hepatic unesterified and esterified retinol. Weanling male Sprague-Dawley rats were allocated to two main diet groups: low iron and controls. After six weeks, plasma retinol concentrations in the low iron groups were reduced >40% compared to the controls. However, of special interest was the observation that the molar ratio of hepatic retinyl esters to retinol was significantly greater in the low iron group compared to the controls,[36] suggesting a vitamin A toxicity state.

The case of an infant was reported who had been given 62,000 IU vitamin A/day for 80 days and showed several clinical signs of retinol intoxication, along with severe anemia and thrombocytopenia. Bone marrow showed a markedly reduced number of erythroid and megakaryocytic cells. Interruption of vitamin A treatment was immediately followed by clinical and biochemical recovery. The authors investigated the activity of retinol on a multipotent hematopoietic cell line and on bone marrow mesenchymal stem cells. Vitamin A strongly inhibited the proliferation of the cells at concentrations similar to those reached in vivo. These were the first findings to demonstrate that infant hypervitaminosis A causes severe anemia and thrombocytopenia, probably due to the direct effect of the molecule on the growth of all bone marrow cellular components.[37]

As noted, anemia is significantly more common in African than European Americans.[22] Laboratory data also indicate the hematocrit, hemoglobin, mean corpuscular volume, serum transferrin saturation and white blood cell counts of African Americans are lower than those of European Americans, but serum ferritin levels are higher.[38] Considering that ferritinemia is associated with increased inflammation,[39] these data collectively support the proposed hypothesis: 1) Rather than deficiencies of either retinol or iron, hemolytic anemia may be due to hypervitaminosis A; 2) People of West Central African descent may be at increased risk of anemia due to sub-clinical hypervitaminosis A, which is controlled by exposure to vitamin A-absorbing endemic parasitemia and by traditional diets, which are low in preformed vitamin A and high in vitamin A-absorbing fiber. In sum, hemolytic anemia may be an indicator of vitamin A toxicity.

Notes

Caring for individuals with sickle cell disease is expensive, with an estimated lifetime cost of $1.7 million per person — which is likely an underestimate. This is due to high costs of care delivered in the emergency department, primarily for severe pain crises when an increased amount of the sickled red blood cells suddenly clump in small blood vessels, the limited access to sickle cell specialists, and the multi-organ dysfunction resulting from this disease. (From "Specialized centers can help realign the U.S.'s moral compass for sickle cell disease" By Amar Kelkar, Julie Kanter and Payal Desai. Dec. 21, 2022, https://www.statnews.com/2022/12/21/realign-moral-compass-sickle-cell-disease/?utm_source=STAT+Newsletters&utm_campaign=c034eff1e3-First_Opinion&utm_medium=email&utm_term=0_8cab1d7961-c034eff1e3-151588037

References

1. WHO South-East Asia. Malaria. https://www.who.int/southeastasia/health-topics/malaria (Accessed January 27, 2023).
2. The Diverse Cuisine of Southeast Asia. https://www.foodnetwork.com/recipes/articles/the-diverse-cuisine-of-southeast-asia (Accessed January 27, 2023).
3. Ranciaro A, Campbell MC, Hirbo JB et al. Genetic origins of lactase persistence and the spread of pastoralism in Africa. Am J Human Genetics 2014; 94(4):496-510. DOI: https://doi.org/10.1016/j.ajhg.2014.02.009
4. Mann GV, Shaffer RD, Anderson RS et al. Cardiovascular disease in the Maasai. Journal Atheroscler Res 1964; 4:289–312. http://www.ncbi.nlm.nih.gov/pubmed/14193818
5. Biss K, Ho KJ, Mikkelson B et al. Some unique biologic characteristics of the Maasai of East Africa. N Engl J Med 1971; 284:694–699. DOI:10.1056/NEJM197104012841304 http://www.ncbi.nlm.nih.gov/pubmed/5107799
6. Wagh K, Bhatia A, Alexe G et al. Lactase persistence and lipid pathway selection in the Maasai. PLOS One 2012; 7(9):e44751. doi:

10.1371/journal.pone.0044751. PMID: 23028602. https://www.wired.com/2012/09/milk-meat-and-blood-how-diet-drives-natural-selection-in-the-maasai/

7. Hanotte O, Bradley DG, Ochieng JW et al. African pastoralism: genetic imprints of origins and migrations. Science 2002; 296:336–339. http://www.ncbi.nlm.nih.gov/pubmed/11951043
8. James WPT, Johnson RJ, Speakman JR et al. Nutrition and its role in human evolution. J Intern Med 2019; 285:533–549.
9. Patel N, Penkert RR, Jones BG, Sealy RE et al. Baseline serum vitamin A and D levels determine benefit of oral vitamin A&D supplements to humoral immune responses following pediatric influenza vaccination. Viruses 2019, 11, 907.
10. Adejumo OE, Kotila TR, Falusi AG et al. Phenotyping and genotyping of CYP2C19 using comparative metabolism of proguanil in sickle-cell disease patients and healthy controls in Nigeria. Pharmacol Res Perspect 2016; 4(5): e00252.
11. Na J, Khan A, Kim JK, Wadood A, Choe YL, Walker DI, Jones DP, Lim CS, Park YH. Discovery of metabolic alterations in the serum of patients infected with Plasmodium spp. by high-resolution metabolomics. Metabolomics. 2019 Dec 23;16(1):9. doi: 10.1007/s11306-019-1630-2. PMID: 31872321.
12. Waugh SM, Willardson BM, Kannan R et al. Heinz bodies induce clustering of band 3, glycophorin, and ankyrin in sickle cell erythrocytes. J Clin Invest 1986; 78(5):1155-60.
13. Luzzatto L, Arese P. Favism and Glucose-6-Phosphate Dehydrogenase deficiency. N Engl J Med 2018; 378:60-71. DOI: 10.1056/NEJMra1708111.
14. Chaves MA, Leonart MS, do Nascimento AJ. Oxidative process in erythrocytes of individuals with hemoglobin S. Hematology 2008; 13(3):187-92. doi: 10.1179/102453308X343356.
15. Hickman MA, Rogers QR, Morris JG. Effect of diet on Heinz body formation in kittens. Am J Vet Res 1990; 51(3):475-8.
16. Whitehead MT, Smitthimedhin A, Webb J et al. Cerebral blood flow and marrow diffusion alterations in children with sickle cell anemia after bone marrow transplantation and transfusion. AJNR Am J Neuroradiol 2018; 39(11):2132-2139. doi: 10.3174/ajnr.A5830.
17. Zhong G, Hogarth C, Snyder JM et al. The retinoic acid hydroxylase Cyp26a1 has minor effects on postnatal Vitamin A homeostasis, but is required for exogenous atRA clearance. J Biol Chem 2019; 294(29):11166-11179.

18. de Oliveira MR. Vitamin A and retinoids as mitochondrial toxicants. Oxid Med Cell Longev 2015; 2015:140267. doi: 10.1155/2015/140267.
19. WHO. Anemia. https://www.who.int/health-topics/anaemia#tab=tab_1 (Accessed January 24, 2023).
20. Ayoya M, Bendech M, Zagré N, Tchibindat F. Maternal anemia in West and Central Africa: Time for urgent action. Public Health Nutrition 2012; 15(5), 916-927. doi:10.1017/S1368980011002424).
21. Joly P, Garnier N, Kebaili K et al. G6PD deficiency and absence of α-thalassemia increase the risk for cerebral vasculopathy in children with sickle cell anemia. Eur J Haematol 2016; 96(4):404-8. doi: 10.1111/ejh.12607.
22. Zakai NA, McClure LA, Prineas R et al. Correlates of anemia in American blacks and whites: the REGARDS Renal Ancillary Study. Am J Epidemiol 2009 Feb 1;169(3):355-64. doi: 10.1093/aje/kwn355. Epub 2008 Dec 9. PMID: 19066309; PMCID: PMC2720717.
23. Semba RD, Bloem MW. The anemia of vitamin A deficiency: epidemiology and pathogenesis. Eur J Clin Nutr 2002; 56, 271–281.
24. Yip R, Dallman PR. Iron. In: Ziegler EE, Filer LJ, editors. Present knowledge in nutrition. 7th ed. Washington DC: ILSI Press; 1996. pp. 278–92.
25. Abbaspour N, Hurrell R, Kelishadi R. Review on iron and its importance for human health. J Res Med Sci. 2014 Feb;19(2):164-74. PMID: 24778671; PMCID: PMC3999603.
26. Staab DB, Hodges RE, Metcalf WK et al. Relationship between vitamin A and iron in the liver. J Nutr 1984; 114(5):840-4. doi: 10.1093/jn/114.5.840. PMID: 6726453.
27. Li Y, Wei CH, Green MH, Ross AC. Dietary iron repletion stimulates hepatic mobilization of vitamin A in previously iron-deficient rats as determined by model-based compartmental analysis. J Nutr 2020; 150(7):1982-1988. doi: 10.1093/jn/nxaa098.
28. Stoffel NU, Zeder C, Brittenham GM, Moretti D, Zimmermann MB. Iron absorption from supplements is greater with alternate day than with consecutive day dosing in iron-deficient anemic women. Haematologica 2020 May;105(5):1232-1239. doi: 10.3324/haematol.2019.220830.)
29. White NJ. What causes malaria anemia? Blood 2022; 139 (15): 2268–2269. doi: https://doi.org/10.1182/blood.2021015055
30. Gkamprela E, Deutsch M, Pectasides D. Iron deficiency anemia in chronic liver disease: etiopathogenesis, diagnosis and treatment. Ann Gastroenterol 2017; 30(4):405-413. doi:10.20524/aog.2017.0152.

31. Ross AC, Owusu SA. Vitamin A metabolism. In Fetal and Neonatal Physiology (Fifth Edition), eds. Polin RA, Abman SH, Fox WW; Saunders, 2011.
32. Dingle T, Lucy JA. Studies on the mode of action of excess vitamin A. The effect of vitamin A on the stability of the erythrocyte membrane. J Biochem 1962; 84:611–21.
33. Urano S, Inomori Y, Sugawara T et al. Vitamin E: inhibition of retinol-induced hemolysis and membrane-stabilizing behavior. J Biol Chem 1992; 267:18365–70.
34. Portolés J, Martín L, Broseta JJ and Cases A (2021) Anemia in Chronic Kidney Disease: From Pathophysiology and Current Treatments, to Future Agents. Front Med 2021; 8:642296. doi: 10.3389/fmed.2021.642296
35. Ono K. Hypervitaminosis A toxicity in regular hemodialysis patients. Trans Am Soc Artif Intern Organs. 1984;30:40-3. PMID: 6543480.
36. Rosales FJ, Jang JT, Piñero DJ et al. Iron deficiency in young rats alters the distribution of vitamin A between plasma and liver and between hepatic retinol and retinyl esters. J Nutr 1999 Jun;129(6):1223-8. doi: 10.1093/jn/129.6.1223.
37. Perrotta S, Nobili B, Rossi F, Criscuolo M, et al. Infant hypervitaminosis A causes severe anemia and thrombocytopenia: evidence of a retinol-dependent bone marrow cell growth inhibition. Blood. 2002 Mar 15;99(6):2017-22. doi: 10.1182/blood.v99.6.2017. PMID: 11877274.)
38. Beutler E, West C. Hematologic differences between African-Americans and whites: the roles of iron deficiency and alpha-thalassemia on hemoglobin levels and mean corpuscular volume. Blood 2005 Jul 15;106(2):740-5. doi: 10.1182/blood-2005-02-0713.
39. Verma N, Chakraverty J, Baweja P, Girotra A et al. Extremely high ferritinemia associated with haemophagocytic lympho histiocytosis (HLH). Indian J Clin Biochem 2017 Mar; 32(1):117-120. doi: 10.1007/s12291-016-0559-8. Epub 2016 Feb 17. PMID: 28149024; PMCID: PMC5247359.

CHAPTER FOURTEEN

CONCLUSIONS

Implications for prevention

The vitamin A toxicity hypothesis of health disparities suggests that the adoption of traditional or modified West Central African-style diets could be studied as an individual and population-based strategy for improving health outcomes both in African Americans and West Central Africans as the latter increasingly adopt western dietary preferences and practices. The plant-based diets of West Central Africa are low in preformed vitamin A and high in vitamin A-absorbing vegetable fiber.[1] Dietary fiber refers to nondigestible carbohydrates and lignin, which are intrinsic and intact in plants, and its consumption lowers the risk of cardiovascular disease, type 2 diabetes, and some cancers.[2] Sources of fiber in these diets are cassava, millet, barley, sorghum, various legumes, fruits, and vegetables.[3] Dietary fiber interacts with the antioxidants in food and interferes with their assimilation. Soluble dietary fiber in the gut reduces the absorption of dietary fats and inhibits the absorption of carotenoids as lipid-soluble compounds.[4] Increased consumption of dietary fiber could therefore contribute importantly to reducing the bioavailability of vitamin A.

The dramatic impact of diet on people of African descent was shown in a study by O'Keefe and colleagues. Twenty African Americans and 20 rural South Africans switched diets for two weeks. The Africans consumed American food, consisting mainly of meat and cheese. The African Americans consumed the African high fiber diet. Africans on the American diet quickly developed intestinal mucosal inflammation and a cytokine profile in the gut related to intestinal cancer. In contrast, when the African Americans were placed on a traditional African diet their existing intestinal inflammation disappeared. In addition, butyrate – a fatty acid known to protect against colon cancer – increased.[5] These effects were interpreted by O'Keefe as suggesting the presence in the US diet of a potential toxin to which people of West Central African descent are especially sensitive. The suggestion here is that the toxin in question is vitamin A.

Testing the theory

Studies needed to test the theory include: 1) comparing vitamin A concentration profiles (serum retinol, retinyl esters, and retinoic acid), the ratio of retinyl esters to total vitamin A, and rates of vitamin A metabolism and catabolism, in healthy African Americans, European Americans, and Americans of other ancestral origins; and 2) comparing vitamin A concentration profiles in African Americans with diseases for which African Americans are at high risk, including organ-specific diseases and conditions. African American patients with these diseases are expected to be more likely than patients with other ancestral backgrounds to have lower concentrations of retinol but increased retinyl ester concentrations, higher percent retinyl esters to total vitamin A, and higher retinoic acid concentrations. African American patients are also predicted to have increased vitamin A levels and expression in the affected tissues, and lower rates of vitamin A metabolism and catabolism. Studies are also indicated, as suggested, to determine the impact of West Central African-style dietary interventions on African American patients with diseases and conditions in which alterations in retinoid profiles are identified.

Conclusions

The centuries-long legacy of enslavement, oppression, and stress suffered by African Americans continues to have pervasive effects, including access to and quality of healthcare and on risks and outcomes of disease. Structural racism and discrimination remain major targets for advocacy, research, and health policy.[6-8] Less well known or well understood is that people of West Central African descent are not only at increased risks of certain diseases but are also at reduced risk of other diseases.[9-11]

The theory has been presented that the overall health of people originally from this region of Africa is related to evolutionary adaptations to the ancestral environment that involved exposure to endemic parasitic organisms and viruses that target the liver. The central challenge of that environment is the major malaria parasite *Plasmodium falciparum,* which selectively absorbs vitamin A from the human host; its use in reproduction is also linked to disease pathogenesis.

The proposed adaptations evolved from natural selection and included 1) sequestering vitamin A away from the liver to other organs, to reduce accessibility to the invaders, and 2) slowing the metabolism and catabolism of vitamin A, causing it to accumulate to subtoxic concentrations and weaken the parasite, thereby reducing disease severity. These adaptations were presumably successful in the original environment and in similar tropical environments. However, in the North American environment characterized by the absence of vitamin A-absorbing parasites and by a dairy-based, vitamin A-rich diet, people of West Central African descent are especially prone to diseases in which vitamin A toxicity is increasingly implicated. Subject to testing, the adoption of a traditional or modified West Central African-style diet, which is low in preformed vitamin A and high in vitamin A-absorbing fiber, could help to prevent and treat these diseases. Subject to testing, it could also serve as a population-based strategy for maintaining overall health and increasing longevity.

References

1. U.S. Department of Agriculture. Trends in U.S. Per Capita Consumption of Dairy Products, 1970-2012 (2014) https://www.ers.usda.gov/amber-waves/2014/june/trendsin-us-per-capita-consumption-of-dairy-products-1970-2012/
2. Dahl WJ, Stewart ML. Position of the Academy of Nutrition and Dietetics: Health Implications of Dietary Fiber. J Acad Nutr Diet 2015; 115:1861-1870. Academy of Nutrition and Dietetics. http://dx.doi.org/10.1016/j.jand.2015.09.003 (Accessed March 25, 2021).
3. O'Keefe SJ, Li JV, Lahti L et al. Fat, fibre and cancer risk in African Americans and rural Africans. Nat Commun 2015 Apr 28;6:6342. doi: 10.1038/ncomms7342. PMID: 25919227; PMCID: PMC4415091.
4. Palafox-Carlos H, Ayala-Zavala JF et al. The role of dietary fiber in the bioaccessibility and bioavailability of fruit and vegetable antioxidants. J Food Sci 2011; 76(1):R6-R15. doi:10.1111/j.1750-3841.2010.01957.x
5. O'Keefe SJ, Li JV, Lahti L et al. Fat, fibre and cancer risk in African Americans and rural Africans. Nat Commun 2015; 6:6342. doi: 10.1038/ncomms7342.
6. Braveman P, Gottlieb L. The social determinants of health: It's time to consider the causes of the causes. Public Health Rep 2014;129(2):19–31.
7. Colen CG, Ramey DM, Cooksey EC et al. Racial disparities in health among nonpoor African Americans and Hispanics: The role of acute and chronic discrimination. Soc Sci Med 2017. pii: S0277-9536(17)30290-3. doi: 10.1016/j.socscimed.2017.04.051.

8. deShazo RD (ed). The Racial Divide in American Medicine: Black Physicians and the Struggle for Justice in Health Care. University Press of Mississippi, Jackson, 2018.
9. Arama C, Skinner J, Doumtabe D, Portugal S et al. Genetic resistance to malaria is associated with greater enhancement of immunoglobulin (Ig)M than IgG responses to a broad array of Plasmodium falciparum antigens. Open Forum Infect Dis. 2015 Aug 26;2(3):ofv118. doi: 10.1093/ofid/ofv118. PMID: 26361633; PMCID: PMC4564391
10. Checkley AM, Smith A, Smith V, Blaze M, et al. Risk factors for mortality from imported falciparum malaria in the United Kingdom over 20 years: an observational study. BMJ. 2012 Mar 27; 344:e2116. doi: 10.1136/bmj.e2116. PMID: 22454091; PMCID: PMC3314185.
11. McGuire RA, Coelho PRP. Slavery and Diseases in the Antebellum American South. In Parasites, Pathogens, and Progress. 2020; 6. Retrieved from https://covid-19.mitpress.mit.edu/pub/8flb6457

OTHER ESSAYS

1

THE PATHOGENESIS OF MALARIA: A NEW PERSPECTIVE

Pathog Glob Health 2013 Apr;107(3):122-9.
doi: 10.1179/2047773213Y.0000000084
The pathogenesis of malaria: a new perspective
Anthony R Mawson
DOI: 10.1179/2047773213Y.0000000084

Abstract

With 3.3 billion people at risk of infection, malaria remains one of the world's most significant health problems. Increasing resistance of the main causative parasite to currently available drugs has created an urgent need to elucidate the pathogenesis of the disease in order to develop new treatments. A possible clue to such understanding is that the malaria parasite *Plasmodium falciparum* selectively absorbs vitamin A from the host and appears to use it for its metabolism; serum vitamin A levels are also reduced in children with malaria. Although vitamin A is essential in low concentration for numerous biological functions, higher concentrations are cytotoxic and prooxidant, and potentially toxic quantities of the vitamin are stored in the liver. During their life cycle in the host the parasites remain in the liver for several days before invading the red blood cells (RBCs). The hypothesis is proposed that the parasites emerge from the liver packed with vitamin A and use retinoic acid (RA), the main biologically active metabolite of vitamin A, as a cell membrane destabilizer to invade the RBCs throughout the body. The characteristic hemolysis and anemia of malaria and other features of the disease may thus be manifestations of an endogenous form of vitamin A intoxication associated with high concentrations of RA but low concentrations of retinol. RA released from the parasites may also affect the fetus and cause preterm birth and fetal growth restriction as a function of the membranolytic and growth inhibitory effects of these compounds, respectively. Subject to testing, the hypothesis suggests that parasite vitamin A metabolism could become a new target for the treatment and prevention of malaria.

Key Words: Malaria; Retinoids; Liver; Parasites; Plasmodium; Anemia; Toxicity; Erythrocyte; Prematurity; Fetal growth restriction; Pathogenesis; Epidemiology

Introduction

About 3.3 billion people – half the world's population – are at risk of malaria due to the main causative parasite, *Plasmodium falciparum. (1)* Over 200 million cases of malaria occur each year, 90% of which occur in Africa, and 655,000 people died from the disease in 2010, making it one of the world's most important health problems. Increasing resistance of the parasite to currently available drugs has created an urgent need to discover new treatments. *(2)* However, this requires an improved understanding of the pathogenesis of malaria. *(3)*

Malarial infection begins when a person is bitten by an infected female anopheles mosquito and Plasmodium spp (species) parasites in the form of sporozoites are injected into the bloodstream. The sporozoites travel to the human liver, multiplying asexually over the next 7-10 days. During this time there are no symptoms. The parasites, now in the form of merozoites, emerge from the liver cells in vesicles and travel through the heart to the capillaries of the lungs. The vesicles eventually disintegrate, freeing the merozoites to enter the bloodstream where they invade and multiply in erythrocytes. When the cells burst, the parasites invade more erythrocytes. Clinical symptoms, including fever, occur in synchrony with the rupture of infected erythrocytes and the release of erythrocyte and parasite debris, including malarial pigment (hemozoin) and glycophosphatidylinositol, the putative "malaria toxin". *(4,5)* In some infected blood cells, instead of replicating asexually, the merozoites develop into sexual forms (gametocytes), which circulate in the bloodstream and are ingested during mosquito bites. The ingested gametocytes develop in the mosquito into mature sex cells (gametes) which develop into ookinetes that actively burrow through the mid-wall of the mosquito and form oocysts, in which develop thousands of active sporozoites. The oocyst eventually bursts, releasing sporozoites that travel to the salivary glands of the mosquito. The cycle of human infection begins again when the mosquito bites another person. *(3)*

The associated features of malaria include severe anemia, fever, thrombocytopenia, chills, headache, vomiting, muscle ache, anorexia, rigor, diarrhea, abdominal discomfort, cough, seizures, respiratory distress, hypoglycemia, metabolic acidosis, hyperlactemia, coma associated with increased intracranial pressure (cerebral malaria), retinopathy, and complications of pregnancy, including preterm birth and low birth weight due to fetal growth restriction. As noted, symptoms are associated with the rupture of infected erythrocytes and the release of putative malaria toxins, which activate peripheral blood mononuclear cells and stimulate the release of cytokines. It is believed that the balance between pro-inflammatory and anti-inflammatory cytokines, chemokines, growth factors and effector molecules determines disease severity. *(6)* Studies have reported increased IL-1B, IL-6, IL-8 and TNF-alpha in late-onset severe disease, and a low IL-10:TNF-alpha ratio. The role of cytokines, however, remains contradictory and unclear. *(3)* Alterations in retinoids (vitamin A and its congeners) also occur in malaria, but the precise role of retinoids in the disease may be different and even opposite to the traditional focus on vitamin A deficiency and supplementation. This paper presents a new theory on the pathogenesis of malaria, suggesting that an endogenous form of hypervitaminosis A induced by the parasite contributes importantly to the signs and symptoms of the disease.

Vitamin A and Malaria

Malaria infection is accompanied by reductions in serum vitamin A concentrations from ≥ 120 mmol/L to ≤ 70 μmol/L (<20 μg/dl), a level usually taken to indicate deficiency in children. *(7)*

In rodent models of malaria there is an inverse correlation between parasitemia and host vitamin A. *(8)* Reduced serum vitamin A levels are also found consistently in children with malaria. *(10)* Such observations have led to the suggestion that *P. falciparum* uses vitamin A from the host for its metabolism; *(11)* in fact, *P. falciparum* selectively absorbs vitamin A from host tissues. This selective uptake of vitamin A was shown by Mizuno et al. *(12)* in a study in which a standard isolate of the parasite was cultured with (3)H-labeled vitamin A at concentrations of the vitamin normally present in human serum. The (3)H-labeled vitamin A accumulated in the parasites in a parasitemia-dependent manner. Radioactivity levels detected in the parasites, found mostly in the cytoplasm, also increased with parasite maturation from the ring to the late trophozoite stage.

Vitamin A supplementation appears to have a protective effect against the disease. For instance, a randomized double-blind, placebo-controlled trial of vitamin A supplementation on morbidity prevention in children in a malaria-endemic area of Papua, New Guinea, showed that supplementation every 3 months for 13 months led to a 30% reduction in the number of confirmed *P. falciparum* febrile episodes compared to the placebo group and a 68% decrease in parasite density. *(13)* A more recent randomized controlled trial on the effect of a single dose of 200,000 IU of vitamin A with daily zinc supplementation for six months on children in Burkina Faso resulted in a significant 30% reduction in slide-confirmed malaria fevers. *(14)* One mechanism suggested for the parasite density-lowering effect is an upregulation of the phagocytotic receptor CD36 and downregulation of cytokines such as TNFα by binding of 9-cis-retinoic acid to the peroxisome proliferator-activated receptor γ (PPARγ) or Retinoid-X-Receptor. *(15)* However, while vitamin A supplementation reduces the incidence of uncomplicated malaria by about one-third, it does not appear to reduce the risk of deaths that can be specifically attributed to malaria. *(10)* The therapeutic potential of vitamin A is also complicated by the fact that retinol antagonizes the antimalarial effect of artemisinin. (*16)* Reversal of the effect of a major drug treatment for malaria suggests that vitamin A may in some way contribute to the disease.

Hamzah et al. *(17)* investigated the role of retinoids as potential antimalarial agents, assessing the effect of all-trans-retinoic acid (RA), 9-cis-RA and 13-cis-RA, as well as retinol itself and its ester, retinyl palmitate, on 3H-hypoxanthine uptake by the laboratory-adapted strains of *P. falciparum*, 3D7 and K1. They also examined the influence of three specific RA receptor antagonists (ER 27191, Ro 41-5253 and AGN 194301) on retinoid-induced growth inhibition of 3D7. All-trans-RA, 9-cis-RA and 13-cis-RA in concentrations ranging from 1 x 10(-4) to 5 x 10(-10) M each had antimalarial activity, but at lesser IC50 values than those of retinol. Retinyl palmitate had minimal effect on 3H-hypoxanthine uptake. Contrary to expectation, each RAR antagonist inhibited 3H-hypoxanthine uptake and demonstrated IC50 values that were comparable to those of retinol. Retinoid antagonists were also weakly antagonistic to the antimalarial effects of retinol.

These complex observations on the role of vitamin A in malaria call for a new perspective on the data. On one hand, *P. falciparum* selectively absorbs vitamin A from the host, low blood concentrations of retinol are associated with severe malaria, and vitamin A supplementation partially protects against malaria infection. These points suggest that vitamin A has an overall beneficial role in malaria. On the other hand, retinol antagonizes the antimalarial effect of artemisinin and retinoid receptor antagonists are as effective as retinol in inhibiting parasite growth, suggesting an opposite role for vitamin A. These apparent contradictions can be resolved if we consider that vitamin A, while essential in low concentration for numerous biological functions, is toxic at higher concentrations; in addition, the merozoite-stage parasite spends several days in the liver, the major storage organ for vitamin A, before invading the erythrocytes. This suggests that serum retinol concentrations are reduced in malaria infection, in part from selective absorption of vitamin A by the parasite, and perhaps to a greater extent from impaired hepatic secretion of vitamin A, since disturbed liver function is recognized in uncomplicated malaria *(18,19)* and especially in severe malaria. *(19)* The absorbed vitamin A, however, may be used by the parasite in ways that contribute to the disease, as suggested below.

Hypothesis of Disease Pathogenesis

Here it is proposed that malaria symptoms are due to an endogenous form of vitamin A intoxication induced by the parasites following their egress from the liver. On this hypothesis, the parasites emerge from the liver packed with vitamin A and use retinoic acid (RA) as a cell membrane destabilizer to invade the red blood cells, causing hemolysis and anemia. Other features of the disease – e.g., fever, headache, muscle aches, gastrointestinal symptoms, seizures, coma, respiratory distress, and retinopathy – may similarly reflect parasite-induced vitamin A toxicity in the brain and other organs, following the transport of RBCs throughout the body and the release of RA (or retinoic acids) into the circulation. It is further suggested that RA released from the parasites also enters the fetus and causes preterm birth and/or intrauterine growth restriction and low birth weight as a function of the membrane destabilizing and growth inhibitory effects of retinoids. This prediction, that low serum retinol concentrations in malaria are accompanied by increased host- and parasite-derived concentrations of RA, has not yet been tested in patients with malaria. If the hypothesis is correct, compounds that alter the metabolism of RA or block its expression may be effective as treatments, not only by attacking the parasite and its nutrition but by blocking the toxic effects of RA released by *P. falciparum* and other Plasmodium species on the human host.

Retinoids

Retinoids (vitamin A and its natural and synthetic congeners) are fat-soluble signaling molecules that are mainly derived from the diet as preformed vitamin A or as provitamin A carotenoids, and are essential for multiple biological functions, including embryonic development, vision, gene expression, tissue differentiation and growth, immune function and mucus secretion. *(20)* Retinoic acid (RA) is produced from free retinol via a process that involves hydrolysis of retinyl esters in the liver, the release of retinol into the circulation and its delivery to the target tissues bound to retinol binding protein (RBP). Retinol is oxidized to retinal (aldehyde) via alcohol dehydrogenase, and RA is synthesized from retinaldehyde via an aldehyde dehydrogenase reaction. RA exerts its effects by binding to and activating two types of nuclear protein receptors: the retinoic acid receptors (RARs) and retinoid X receptors (rexinoids, RXRs), both of which exist as three distinct gene products (alpha, beta and gamma). These receptors control the expression of numerous target genes by binding to specific DNA sequences termed RA response elements (RAREs). *(21,22)* About 90% of body stores of vitamin A are contained in the liver, in quantities sufficient to last the average adult about two years without the need for additional intake. *(23)* Serum retinol levels remain stable due to a carefully regulated transport system that ensures the target tissues receive the necessary amounts of retinol despite major fluctuations in dietary intake. *(24)*

While retinoids in low concentrations act as growth factors, higher concentrations are prooxidant, cytotoxic, mutagenic and teratogenic, especially when unbound to protein. Vitamin A toxicity is due mainly to excessive dietary intake or to self-medication, when the liver becomes saturated with vitamin A and stored retinyl esters spill over into the circulating blood. Retinyl esters react more randomly with cell membranes than the physiologically-sequestered RBP and hence are a major form of vitamin A toxicity. *(25,26)* Large single or short-term doses of preformed vitamin A can induce a condition of acute toxicity characterized by nausea, vomiting, headache, fatigue, vertigo, blurred vision, increased intracranial pressure, irritability and lack of muscular coordination. The symptoms of chronic vitamin A poisoning are varied and can be manifested by central nervous system effects, liver abnormalities, growth arrest in children, bone and skin changes, and other adverse effects. Even low intakes of vitamin A in early pregnancy (7,800 μg/day) are associated with congenital malformations. *(27)* Retinoid toxicity can also occur in cholestasis, when the secretion of retinol-binding protein is inhibited, vitamin A accumulates in the liver, and biliary material (including metabolites of retinol, retinyl acetate, retinal or retinoic acid) spills over into the circulation and is reabsorbed. *(28)*

Possible Role of Retinoid Toxicity in Malaria Pathogenesis

Clinical manifestations of severe falciparum malaria typically include severe anemia and respiratory distress. Anemia is the primary clinical manifestation of severe malaria in children, with mortality rates that can exceed 30% among children under five years of age. Asexual blood stage parasites produce 8-20 new merozoites every 48 hours, causing parasite numbers to increase rapidly to levels as high as 10 trillion (10^{13}) per host. *(29)* Host cell invasion is controlled by the sequential secretion of proteins from two types of specialized organelles: micronemes and rhoptries. *(30,31)* The pathophysiological processes that contribute to severe anemia include destruction of parasitized and nonparasitized red blood cells, inefficient or suppressed erythropoiesis, and dyserythropoiesis associated with impaired innate immunity. *(3)* However, the precise mechanisms responsible for parasite entry, which requires localized destabilization of the host cytoskeleton and takes place in a matter of seconds, are unknown. *(32)*.

It is hypothesized that the signs and symptoms of malaria are due to the effects of vitamin A accumulated by the parasites in the host liver. It is proposed that the parasites use the vitamin A, in the form of retinoic acid, to invade the RBCs; RA is then distributed via the transport of RBCs throughout the body in toxic concentrations. On this hypothesis, *hemolysis and anemia* are due to the membranolytic actions of RA released from the parasites to invade the RBCs. Retinoids, including retinol and RA, can inhibit cell growth and interact directly with membranes to increase their permeability and fluidity, causing hemolysis of erythrocytes and increased secretion of enzymes from lysosomes. *(33)* Cells exposed briefly to retinol show marked swelling, while longer exposures cause cell death; cultured human lymphoblastoid cells exposed to retinol and retinoic acid undergo a time- and dose-dependent decrease in viability accompanied by cell swelling. (*34)* Retinoids also arrest the growth of cultured lymphocytes due to a membrane destabilizing effect. (*35)* Retinol-induced erythrocyte hemolysis appears to be caused by physical damage to the membrane micelle induced by penetration of retinol molecules rather than by oxidative disruption of erythrocyte membrane lipids initiated by retinol oxidation. (*36)* RA fosters the phagocytosis of parasitized erythrocytes, which is stimulated by phosphatidylserine exposure at the cell surface. Exposure to RA and a specific RAR agonist, 4-(E-2-[5,6,7,8-tetrahydro-5,5,8,8-tetramethyl-2-naphthalenyl]-1-propenyl) benzoic acid (TTNPB), significantly increased erythrocyte annexin binding, an effect reflecting cell shrinkage, and significantly increased cytosolic Ca(2+)-activity, a known trigger of phosphatidylserine exposure. Infection of erythrocytes with *P. falciparum* also increased phosphatidylserine exposure, an effect that was facilitated by the presence of TTNPB. *(37)*

The fact that RA and TTNPB trigger phosphatididylserine exposure and cell shrinkage of erythrocytes, which are typical features of suicidal erythrocyte death or eryptosis, supports the present hypothesis that the malaria parasite itself uses RA accumulated in the host liver to invade erythrocytes. Other signs and symptoms may be similarly due to generalized and localized endogenous forms of host- and parasite-generated vitamin A poisoning in the affected tissues:

- Fever, fatigue and malaise may represent generalized, nonspecific effects of retinoid toxicity, as seen in the retinoic acid syndrome associated with the use of retinoic acid (13-cis-retinoic acid or isotretinoin) as a treatment for acute promyelocytic leukemia. *(38)*
- Respiratory distress associated with interstitial pulmonary infiltrates, pleural and pericardial effusion and dyspnea is seen in over 80% of patients with the retinoic acid syndrome. (*38)*
- Thrombocytopenia, one of the most common complications of severe malaria, (*39)* is also a feature of hypervitaminosis A. For instance, hypervitaminosis A in infants causes severe thrombocytopenia and anemia, which appears to be due to a direct inhibitory effect on the growth of all bone marrow cellular components and may be mediated by the up-regulation of cyclin-dependent kinase inhibitors. (*40)*
- Headache and intracranial hypertension in malaria may be equivalent to pseudotumor cerebri (PTC), a feature of acute hypervitaminosis A. (*41)*
- Retinopathy and papilledema in malaria could also be associated with hypervitaminosis A. Exposure to isotretinoin can cause retinopathy and optic nerve abnormalities, *(42)* and RA contributes to light-induced retinopathy in mice via plasma membrane permeability and mitochondrial poisoning, leading to caspase activation and mitochondria-associated cell death. (*43)*
- Malaria in pregnancy contributes to a substantial number of maternal deaths as well as infant deaths resulting from preterm birth, fetal growth restriction (FGR) and low birth weight. (*44)* The present hypothesis suggests that retinoids released from the parasites enter the fetus and cause preterm birth and/or FGR and subsequent low birth weight due to the membranolytic and growth-inhibiting effects of excess circulating retinoids, respectively. This hypothesis is supported by the results of a study by the author and colleagues using an animal model of preeclampsia, in which severe gestational diabetes and fetal growth restriction (FGR) were induced by the drug streptozotocin.*(45)* In this study, FGR was associated with markedly increased liver enzymes and alterations in retinoid profiles suggesting retinoid toxicity, e.g., the percentage of retinyl esters as a

fraction of total vitamin A, normally < 10%, *(25)* was 23% versus 11% in the untreated control group. The ratio of retinyl esters to retinol and the concentration of RA were also significantly increased compared to control values. If the present hypothesis is correct, the putative malaria toxin could be retinoic acid or a related metabolite of vitamin A.

Further Implications of the Retinoid Toxicity Hypothesis for Malaria

In mice made moderately diabetic with streptozotocin, infection with *P. yoelli* malaria or injection of extracts from malaria-parasitized RBCs has been found to normalize the associated hyperglycemia. *(46)* There is growing evidence of an association between type 2 diabetes mellitus and alterations in retinoid metabolism, including an increase in circulating RBP, the transport protein for retinol; moreover, exercise lowers the concentration of retinoid and improves glucose metabolism. *(47,48)* The present hypothesis suggests that the normalization of hyperglycemia in malaria-infected diabetic mice is due to the selective absorption of vitamin A by the parasites and its reduction below a critical threshold.

Co-infection with helminths also protects against severe malaria. *(49,50)* This may be tentatively explained on the present hypothesis as follows. The parasitic worm *Onchocerciasis volvulus,* like *P. falciparum*, selectively absorbs and concentrates vitamin A, such that the retinol concentration in *O.volvulus* is about eight times higher than that in the surrounding tissues of the host. *(51)* The present hypothesis suggests that *O. volvulus* reduces the availability of vitamin A for the malaria parasite in the early sporozoite or blood stage of the lifecycle, which starves and weakens the parasite, perhaps reducing the numbers of parasites reaching the liver and thereby lessening symptom severity.

How Does the Merozoite Avoid the Host Immune System?

The merozoite stage of the malaria parasite lifecycle begins within host hepatocytes. The merozoites reach the circulation via hepatic sinusoids, followed by erythrocyte invasion and the appearance of disease symptoms. *(52)* The mechanism by which the merozoites escape the host immune system before erythrocyte invasion is unknown. Using a mouse model of malaria, Sturm et al. *(53)* showed that the parasites kill and detach their host hepatocytes, after which parasite-filled vesicles (merosomes) emerge into the sinusoidal lumen. The parasites simultaneously inhibit the release of phosphatidyl serine (PS) onto the outer leaflet of the host plasma membrane, which enhances phagocytosis. Thus, hepatocyte-derived merosomes ensure both the migration of parasites into the blood stream and their protection from host immunity.

On the present hypothesis, this process may be due to the uptake of hepatic retinol by the parasites, followed by the localized release of high concentrations of retinoic acid or other polar metabolites, causing the destruction of host hepatocytes and the simultaneous depletion of retinoid in surrounding host cells, leading to loss of potency of immune system defense mechanisms. Sturm *et al.* *(53)* reported that host cell death did not occur by classical necrosis or apoptosis but by activation of cysteine proteases. This was suggested by the observation that treatment of infected hepatocytes with the cysteine protease inhibitor E64 completely inhibited parasitophorus vacuole membrane (PVM) destruction and cytochrome c release. Examination of infected hepatocytes early after detachment revealed condensation of the cell nuclei, suggesting that cell death was occurring. This was supported by loss of mitochondrial membrane potential, the release of cytochrome c from the mitochondria of infected cells, and alterations in the shape of the mitochondria. Consistent with the retinoid hypothesis, all-trans RA disturbs mitochondrial function long before detectable signs of cell death. *(54)* It was also noted that, like *P. falciparum* erythrocyte merozoites, hepatic merozoites actively accumulate intracellular Ca^{2+} released from damaged stores of dying host to higher levels than those of host cells. This process could be one aspect of the selective uptake of retinoid by the parasite from surrounding host cells, since cellular calcium homeostasis interacts with signaling systems involved in the control of retinoic acid-dependent transcriptional activity. *(55)* The observation that early Plasmodium liver stages confer resistance to apoptosis to the host cell *(56)* could be related to the active depletion of retinol in those cells by the parasite. Indeed, dead parasites do not protect host cells from undergoing cell death. *(57)* In summary, it is postulated that the process by which Plasmodium liver stage parasites manipulate their host cells to ensure the safe delivery of merozoites into the blood stream is related to alterations in host retinoid metabolism and immunity induced by selective retinoid uptake and release by the parasite.

Implications of the Model for Understanding Current Treatments

Low levels of arginine, the precursor for nitric oxide (NO), are common in patients with malaria and are associated with endothelial dysfunction.

Administering arginine intravenously reverses hypoargininemia and endothelial dysfunction. Carbon monoxide shares certain functional properties with NO and protects against cerebral malaria in mice. Arginine therapy may therefore prove beneficial in severe malaria in addition to conventional antimalarial treatment. *(58)* Consistent with the retinoid toxicity hypothesis, the potential efficacy of NO in the treatment of malaria could be due to the fact that RA and NO are inversely related; *(45)* hypoargininemia could therefore reflect increased RA. This suggests that arginine or NO therapy could be effective in malaria by inhibiting the actions of RA.

The quinolines (including chloroquine, primaquine, mefloquine and quinine) are among the most successful yet poorly understood classes of drugs, with important uses in the treatment of systemic lupus erythematosus and HIV as well as malaria. The 8-amino-quinolines such as primaquine and tafenoquine are the only drugs that target the liver stage malaria parasites. *(29)* The therapeutic effectiveness of these drugs may lie in their ability to affect vitamin A metabolism, specifically by inhibiting the conversion of retinol to retinoic acid, the latter of which may be critical for the nutrition of the malaria parasite, as well as by increasing retinol to concentrations that are toxic to the parasites. At noted, RA is produced from the oxidation of retinol to retinal via the action of an alcohol dehydrogenase, and from retinaldehyde via an aldehyde dehydrogenase reaction. Thus, the quinolines may be acting as dehydrogenase inhibitors. This is supported by the fact that aldehyde dehydrogenase 1 (ALDH1) is selectively inhibited by quinolones; other known inhibitors of ALDH1 are also lethal to or inhibit the growth of *P. falciparum* in vitro. *(60)*

Implications for New Treatments

The treatment of malaria currently depends on few available compounds, and these are vulnerable to the emergence of compound-resistant parasites and mosquitoes. *(29)* Subject to obtaining positive results based on tests of the proposed model, new treatments for malaria could be developed using agents that target the metabolism or expression of retinoids. Such treatments would be expected to eliminate the parasite by affecting its nutritional status as well as treating the manifestations of the disease, i.e., by inhibiting the clinical effects of host- and parasite-derived retinoic acid.

With regard to alternative treatments suggested by the hypothesis, a randomized, double-blind, placebo-controlled phase I/II trial of rosiglitazone, a peroxisome proliferator-activated receptor gamma (PPARγ) agonist (4 mg twice daily for 4 days), showed that the drug significantly enhanced parasite clearance times compared with controls. Rosiglitazone also reduced inflammatory biomarkers to malaria infection and was described as well-tolerated as an adjunct to standard therapy for nonsevere *P. falciparum* malaria. *(61)* Several studies indicate that PPARγ ligands regulate differentiation and induce cell growth arrest and apoptosis in a variety of cancer types. *(62)* It is of special interest that the first RARα antagonist to be developed, Ro41-5253, *(63)* is a PPARγ agonist in that it binds and activates PPARγ, albeit weakly. *(64)* This suggests that expression of PPARy is effectively equivalent to RARα antagonism and the latter is a natural consequence of PPARγ activation or expression. These observations support the retinoid toxicity hypothesis and suggest that RAR antagonists themselves could be useful in the treatment of malaria.

Other compounds with anti-retinoid actions could be explored as potential treatments for malaria. For instance, the cytolytic effects of retinol on biological membranes are counteracted by tocopherol, which may act as a membrane stabilizer through interaction with polyunsaturated fatty acid residues of phospholipid molecules. *(65)* The presence of tocopherol (200 microM) as well as taurine (5-20 mM) and zinc (50-100 microM) were reported to protect cultured human lymphoblastoid cells from retinol-induced injury, and the combination of all three compounds afforded complete protection, possibly though a membrane stabilizing action unrelated to lipid peroxidation. *(34)* Taurine, zinc, and tocopherol could be tested together as anti-malarial agents, as well as in combination with RAR antagonists.

The retinoid toxicity hypothesis has implications for the development of malaria vaccines, development of which has been hampered by an incomplete understanding of the pathogenesis of the disease; in particular, uncertainty regarding the immunological processes that provide protection after vaccination with irradiated sporozoites. *(66)* Immunity from severe malaria is acquired rapidly, after only 1-2 episodes of severe disease. *(67)* Given that vitamin A can function as an adjuvant, i.e., by promoting vaccine antibody responses, *(68)* it is possible that vitamin A supplementation functions as a vaccine or vaccine adjuvant in malaria, "inoculating" the host from the presumably more toxic "dose" of retinoid from the parasite by prior exposure to a lesser dose. Studies showing that vitamin A partially protects against malaria infection *(9,10)* could therefore be interpreted as indicating that, in this role, vitamin A functions as a vaccine adjuvant rather than as a nutritional supplement to prevent vitamin A deficiency. The mechanism of adjuvant action may involve feedback inhibition of the production of vitamin A, since administered RA can inhibit the endogenous synthesis of

RA. For instance, Barua et al. *(69)* found that a single oral dose of RA (0.167 mM) in corn oil given to 6 healthy human subjects led to a mean decline in serum retinol (ROL) of approximately 20% within 1 hour and lasted for 24 hours.

Guilbride *(70)* has proposed that malaria vaccines fail because of live parasites in the skin and the presence of regulatory T cells (Tregs), which inhibit the immune response and block vaccine function. The retinoid toxicity hypothesis suggests that Tregs are activated in the skin of patients with malaria due to high concentrations of RA released by the parasites. In support of this suggestion, RA enhances the de novo differentiation of naïve CD4+ cells to Foxp3+ Tregs and suppresses Th17 development. *(71)*

It remains for future work to explore the theoretical and practical implications of these concepts. In the meantime, the present hypothesis could be tested initially by determining whether, as predicted, low serum concentrations of retinol are associated with high concentrations of retinoic acid both in animal models and in patients with malaria compared to noninfected controls. Subject to the outcomes of such tests, parasite retinoid metabolism could become a new target for the treatment and prevention of malaria.

References

1. WHO. *World Malaria Report 2008*. Geneva, Switzerland: WHO, (2008).
2. J. Crawley, C. Chu, G. Mtove, F. Nosten. Malaria in children. *Lancet* **375**, 1468-1481 (2010).
3. D. J. Perkins, T. Were, G. C. Davenport, P. Kempaiah, J. B. Hittner. Severe malarial anemia: innate immunity and pathogenesis. *Int J Biol Sci* **7,** 1427-1442 (2011).
4. L. Schofield L, F. Hackett F. Signal transduction in host cells by a glycophosphatidylinositol toxin of malaria parasites. *J Exp Med* 1993; **177**:145-153.
5. I. A. Clark, W. B. Cowden. The pathophysiology of falciparum malaria. *Pharmacol Ther* **99**, 221-260 (2003).
6. J. Langhorne, F.M. Ndungu, A.M. Sponaas, K. Marsh. Immunity to malaria: more questions than answers. *Nat Immunol* 2008; **9**:1145-1152.
7. International Vitamin A Consultative Group*: A Brief Guide to Current Methods Assessing Vitamin A Status.* Washington, DC: The Nutrition Foundation; 1993.

8. F. J. Rosales, J. D.Topping, J. E. Smith, A. H. Shankar, A. C. Ross. Relation of serum retinol to acute phase proteins and malarial morbidity in Papua New Guinea children. *Am J Clin Nutr* **71**, 1582–1588 (2000).
9. S. Müller, B. Kappes. Vitamin and cofactor biosynthesis pathways in Plasmodium and other apicomplexan parasites. *Trends Parasitol* **23,** (3):112-21 (2007).
10. M.A. SanJoaquin, M.E. Molyneux. Malaria and vitamin A deficiency in African children: a vicious circle? *Malaria J* **8**, 134 doi:10.1186/1475-2875-8-134 (2009).
11. I. Gouado, L. G. Lehman, I. T. Some, Y. Mbouyap, M. J. B. Pankoui, A. R. Ejoh, M. F. Tchouanguep. Influence of malaria on the serum levels of vitamin A, zinc and calcium of children in Doula-Cameroon. *Afr J Biotechnol* **6**, 871-876 (2007).
12. Y. Mizuno, S. I. Kawazu, S. Kano, N. Watanabe, T. Matsuura, et al. In-vitro uptake of vitamin A by Plasmodium falciparum. *Ann Trop Med Parasitol* **97**, 237-43 (2003).
13. A.H. Shankar, B. Genton, R.D. Semba, M. Baisor, J. Paino, S. Tamja, T. Adiguma, L. Wu, L. Rare, J.M. Tielsch, M.P. Alpers, K.P. West Jr. Effect of vitamin A supplementation on morbidity due to Plasmodium falciparum in young children in Papua New Guinea: a randomised trial. *Lancet* **354,** 203–209 (1999).
14. A.N. Zeba, H. Sorgho, N. Rouamba, I. Zongo, J. Rouamba, R.T. Guiguemde, D.H. Hamer, N. Mokhtar, J.B. Ouedraogo. Major reduction of malaria morbidity with combined vitamin A and zinc supplement in young children in Burkina Faso: a randomized double blind trial. *Nutrition J* **7**, 7 (2008).
15. L. Serghides, K. C. Kain. Mechanism of protection induced by vitamin A in falciparum malaria. Lancet **359**, 1404–1406 (2002).
16. T. Skinner-Adams, H. Barrett, T.M. Davis. Heterogeneous activity in vitro of vitamin A (retinol) in combination with novel and established antimalarial drugs. Trans R Soc Trop Med Hyg **93**, 550-1 (1999).
17. J. Hamzah, T. S. Skinner-Adams, T. M. Davis. In vitro antimalarial activity of retinoids and the influence of selective retinoic acid receptor antagonists. *Acta Trop* **87**, 345-53 (2003).
18. M.P. Grobusch, P.G. Kremsner. Uncomplicated malaria. *Curr Top Microbiol Immunol* **295,** 83-104 (2005).
19. A. Bhalla, V. Suri, V. Singh. Malarial hepatopathy. *J Postgrad Med* **52**(4), 315-20 (2006).
20. D.N. D'Ambrosio, R.D. Clugston, W.S. Blaner. Vitamin A metabolism: an update. *Nutrients* **3**(1), 63-103 (2011).

21. G. Litwack, editor. *Vitamin A: Vitamins and Hormones*, Vol. 75. San Diego, CA: Elsevier Academic Press (2007).
22. M. Theodosiou, V. Laudet, M. Schubert. From carrot to clinic: an overview of the retinoic acid signaling pathway. *Cell Mol Life Sci* **67**, 1423-45 (2010).
23. L.M. De Luca, K.E. Creek. Vitamin A and the liver. *Prog Liver Dis* **8**, 81-98 (1986).
24. R. Blomoff, H. K. Blomhoff. Overview of retinoid metabolism and function. *J Neurobiol* **66**, 606-630 (2006).
25. K. L. Penniston, S. A. Tanumihardjo. The acute and chronic toxic effects of vitamin A. *Am J Clin Nutr* **83**, 191-201 (2006).
26. M. R. De Oliveira, R. F. Da Rocha, M. A. Pasquali, J. C. Moreira. The effects of vitamin A supplementation for 3 months on adult rat nigrostriatal axis: increased monoamine oxidase enzyme activity, mitochondrial redox dysfunction, increased β-amyloid(1-40) peptide and TNF-α contents, and susceptibility of mitochondria to an in vitro H2O2 challenge. *Brain Res Bull* **87**, 432-44 (2012).
27. L.H. Allen LH, M. Haskell M. Estimating the potential for vitamin A toxicity in women and young children. *J Nutr* **132**, 2907S-2919S (2002).
28. M. A. Leo, Lieber CS. Hypervitaminosis A: A liver lover's lament. *Hepatology* **8**, 412-417 (1988).
29. B. M. Greenwood, D. A. Fidock, D. E. Kyle, S. H. I. Kappe, P. L. Alonso, F. H. Collins, P. E. Duffy. Malaria: progress, perils and prospects for eradication. *J Clin Invest* **118**, 1266-1276 (2008).
30. V. B. Carruthers, F. M. Tomley. Receptor-ligand interaction and invasion: microneme proteins in apicomplexans. *Subcell Biochem* **47**, 33-45 (2008).
31. J. M. Santos, D. Soldati-Favre. Invasion factors are coupled to key signaling events leading to the establishment of infection in apicomplexan parasites. *Cell Microbiol* **13**, 787 (2011).
32. S. Besteiro, J. F. Dubremetz, M. Lebrun. The moving junction of apicomplexan parasites: a key structure for invasion. *Cell Microbiol* **13**, 797-805 (2011).
33. T. Dingle, J. A. Lucy. Studies on the mode of action of excess vitamin A. The effect of vitamin A on the stability of the erythrocyte membrane. *J. Biochem* **84**, 611-621 (1962)
34. H. Pasantes-Morales, C.E. Wright, G. E. Gaull. Protective effect of taurine, zinc and tocopherol on retinol-induced damage in human lymphoblastoid cells. *J Nutr* **114,** 2256-2261 (1984).

35. I. Gery. Inhibition of DNA and RNA synthesis in lymphocyte cultures by rod outer segments and its counteraction by vitamin E and other antioxidants. *Invest Ophthalmol* **19**, 751-759 (1980).
36. S. Urano, Y. Inomori, T. Sugawara, Y. Kato, M. Kitahara, et al. Vitamin E: inhibition of retinol-induced hemolysis and membrane-stabilizing behavior. *J Biol Chem* **267**, 18365 (1992).
37. O. M. Niemoeller, M. Foller, C. Lang, S.M. Huber, F. Lang. Retinoic acid induced suicidal erythrocyte death. *Cell Physiol Biochem* **21**(1-3), 193-202 (2008).
38. E. Patatanian, D. F. Thompson. Retinoic acid syndrome: a review. *J Clin Pharm Ther* **33**, 331-8 (2008).
39. M. V. Lacerda, M.P. Mourão MP, H. C. Coelho, J. B. Santos. Thrombocytopenia in malaria: who cares? *Mem Inst Oswaldo Cruz* **106**, (Suppl 1), 52-63 (2011).
40. S. Perrotta, B. Nobili, F. Rossi, M. Crisuolo, A. Iolascon, et al. Infant hypervitaminosis A causes severe anemia and thrombocytopenia: evidence of a retinol-dependent bone marrow cell growth inhibition. *Blood* **99**, 2017-22 (2008).
41. B. Machner, B. Neppert, M. Paulsen, C. Hofmann, T. Sander. Pseudotumor cerebri as a reversible side effect of all-trans retinoic acid treatment in acute promyelocytic leukaemia. *Eur J Neurol* **15**, (7):e68-9 (2008).
42. E.J. Lammer, D. T. Chen, R. M. Hoar, N. D. Agnish, P. J. Benke, J. T. Braun, C. J. Curry, P. M. Fernhoff, A. W. Grix, Jr., I. T. Lott, et al. Retinoic acid embryopathy. *N Engl J Med* **313,** 837-41 (1985).
43. A. Maeda, T. Maeda, M. Golczak, S. Chou, A. Desai. Involvement of all-trans-retinal in acute light-induced retinopathy of mice. *J Biol Chem* **284**, 15173-83 (2009).
44. M. Desai, F. O. Ter Kuile, F. O. Nosten, R. McGready, K. Asamoa, *et al*. Epidemiology and burden of malaria in pregnancy. *Lancet Infect Dis* **7**, 93-104 (2007).
45. A.R. Mawson, W. Bennett, S. Tanumihardjo, J. Mills, A. Smith, P. Kirui, W. May, J.N. Martin JN Jr. Altered retinoid profiles in an animal model of preeclampsia, gestational diabetes and fetal growth restriction. *Reprod Sci* **17** (3), 235A; Supplement: Abstract 592 (2010).
46. K.M. Elased, K.A. Gumaa, J.B. de Souza, H. H. Rahmoune, J.H. Playfair, T.W. Rademacher. Reversal of type 2 diabetes in mice by products of malaria parasites. II. Role of inositol phosphoglycans (IPGs). *Mol Genet Metab* **73**(3), 248-58 (2001).
47. T.E. Graham, Q. Yang, M. Blüher, A. Hammarstedt, T.P. Ciaraldi, R.R. Henry, C.J. Wason, A. Oberbach, P.A Jansson, U. Smith, B.B. Kahn.

Retinol-binding protein 4 and insulin resistance in lean, obese, and diabetic subjects. *N Engl J Med* **354**(24):2552-63 (2006).
48. J.M. Starkey, Y. Zhao, R.G. Sadygov, S.J. Haidacher, W.S. Lejeune, N. Dey, B.A. Luxon, M.A. Kane, J.L. Napoli, L. Denner, R.G. Tilton. Altered retinoic acid metabolism in diabetic mouse kidney identified by O isotopic labeling and 2D mass spectrometry. *PLoS One* **5**(6):e11095 (2010).
49. T. W. Mwanga, J. M. Bethony, S. Brooker. Malaria and helminth interactions in humans: an epidemiological viewpoint. *Ann Trop Med Parasitol* **100**, 551-570 (2006).
50. F. C. Hartgers, M. Yazdanbakhsh. Co-infection of helminths and malaria: modulation of the immune responses to malaria. *Parasite Immunol* **28**, 497-506 (2006).
51. D. Stürchler, D. Wyss, A. Hanck. Retinol, onchocerciasis and *Onchocerca volvulus*. *Trans Roy Soc Trop Med Hyg* **75**, 617 (1981).
52. U. Frevert, S. Engelmann, S. Zoubédé, J. Stange, B. Ng, et al. Intravital observation of *Plasmodium berghei* sporozoite infection of the liver. *PLoS Biol* **3,** (6):e192 (2005).
53. A. Sturm, R. Amino, C. van de Sand, T. Regen, S. Retzlaff. Manipulation of host hepatocytes by the malaria parasite for delivery into liver sinusoids. *Science* **313,** 1287-90 (2006).
54. J. Schmidt-Wende, V. Gogvadze, E. Hellstrom-Lindberg, B. Zhivotsky. Early mitochondrial alterations in ATRA-induced cell death. *Cell Death Differ* **13**, 119-128. (2006).
55. S. Launay, M. Gianni, L. Diomede, L. M. Machesky, J. Enouf, B. Papp. Enhancement of ATRA-induced cell differentiation by inhibition of calcium accumulation into the endoplasmic retinulum: cross-talk between RAR alpha and calcium-dependent signaling. *Blood* **101**, 3220-8 (2003).
56. P. Leiriao, S. S. Albuquerque, S. Corso, G. J. Van Gemert, R. W. Sauerwein, et al. HGF/MET signalling protects Plasmodium-infected host cells from apoptosis. *Cell Microbiol* **7**, 603-9 (2005).
57. C. Van de Sand, S. Horstmann, A. Schmidt, A. Sturm, S. Bolte, et al. The liver stage of Plasmodium berghei inhibits host cell apoptosis. *Mol Microbiol_* **58**, (3):731-42 (2005).
58. J.B.Weinberg, B.K. Lopansri, E. Mwaikambo, D.L. Granger. Arginine, nitric oxide, carbon monoxide, and endothelial function in severe malaria. *Curr Opin Infect Dis* **21**(5), 468-75 (2008).
59. A. Sirsjö A, A.C. Gidlöf AC, A. Olsson A, H. Törmä H, M. Ares M, H. Kleinert H, U.Förstermann U, G.K. Hansson GK. Retinoic acid inhibits

nitric oxide synthase-2 expression through the retinoic acid receptor-alpha. *Biochem Biophys Res Commun* **270**(3):846-51 (2000).
60. P. R. Graves, J. J. Kwiek, P. Fadden, et al. Discovery of novel targets of quinoline drugs in the human purine binding proteome. *Mol Pharmacol* **62**, 1364-1372 (2002).
61. A. K. Boggild, S. Krudsood, S. N. Patel, L. Serghides, N. Tangpukdee, *et al.* Use of peroxisome proliferator-activated receptor gamma agonists as adjunctive treatment for *Plasmodium falciparum* malaria: a randomized, double-blind, placebo-controlled trial. *Clin Infect Dis* **49,** 841-9 (2009).
62. A. Papi, P. Rocchi, A. M. Ferreri, F. Guerra, M. Orlandi. Enhanced effects of PPARγ ligands and RAR selective retinoids in combination to inhibit migration and invasiveness in cancer cells. *Oncol Rep* **21**, 1083-1089 (2009).
63. C. Apfel, F. Bauer, M. Crettaz, L. Forni, M. Kamber, et al. A retinoic acid receptor alpha antagonist selectively counteracts retinoic acid effects. Proc *Natl Acad Sci U S A* **89**, 7129–7133 (1992).
64. M. Schupp, J. C. Curtin, R. J. Kim, A. N. Billin, M. A. Lazar. A widely used retinoic acid receptor antagonist induces peroxisome proliferator-activated receptor-γ activity. *Mol Pharmacol* **71**, 1251-1257 (2007).
65. J. B. Massey, H. S. She, H. J. Pownall. Interaction of vitamin E with saturated phospholipid bilayers. *Biochem Biophys Res Commun* **106**, 842-847 (1982).
66. S. L. Hoffman, L. M. Goh, T. C. Luke, I. Schneider, T. P. Le, D. L. Doolan, J. Sacci, P. de la Vega, M. Dowler, C. Paul, D. M. Gordon, J. A. Stoute, L. W. Church, M. Sedegah, D. G. Heppner, W. R. Ballou, T. L. Richie. Protection of humans against malaria by immunization with radiation-attenuated Plasmodium falciparum sporozoites. *J Infect Dis* **185,** (8):1155-64 (2002).
67. S. Gupta, R.W. Snow, C.A. Donnelly, K. Marsh, C. Newbold. Immunity to non-cerebral severe malaria is acquired after one or two infections. *Nat Med* **5** (3):340-3 (1999).
68. A. C. Ross. Vitamin A supplementation and retinoic acid treatment in the regulation of antibody responses in vivo. *Vitam Horm* **75**, 197-222 (2007).
69. A.B. Barua, P.K. Duitsman, D. Kostic, M. Barua, J.A. Olson. Reduction of serum retinol levels following a single oral dose of all-trans retinoic acid in humans. *Int J Vitam Nutr Res* **67**, 423-6 (1997).
70. D. L. Guilbride, P. Gawlinski, P. D. Guilbride. Why functional pre-erythrocytic and bloodstage malaria vaccines fail: a meta-analysis of

fully protective immunizations and novel immunological model. *PLoS One* **5,** e10685 (2010).

71. X. Zhou, N. Kong, J. Wang, H. Fan, H. Zou, *et al.* Cutting edge: all-trans retinoic acid sustains the stability and function of natural regulatory T cells in an inflammatory milieu. *J Immunol* **185**, 2675-9 (2010).

Note

The retinoid toxicity hypothesis of malaria has been tested in one study and was confirmed:

From the Abstract:

Metabolic interactions between the host and Plasmodium may present novel targets for malaria control, but such interactions are yet to be deciphered. An exploration of metabolic interactions between humans and two Plasmodium species by high-resolution metabolomics may provide fundamental insights that can aid the development of a new strategy for the control of malaria. Objectives: This study aimed at exploring the metabolic changes in the sera of patients infected with Plasmodium falciparum and Plasmodium vivax. Methods: Uni- and multivariate metabolomic analyses were performed on the sera of four groups of patients, namely normal control (N, n = 100), P. falciparum-infected patients (PF, n = 21), P. vivax-infected patients (PV, n = 74), and non-malarial pyretic patients (Pyr, n = 25). Results: Univariate and multivariate analyses of N, PF, and PV groups showed differential metabolic phenotypes and subsequent comparisons in pairs revealed significant features. Pathway enrichment test with significant features showed the affected pathways, namely glycolysis/gluconeogenesis for PF and retinol metabolism for PV. The metabolites belonging to the affected pathways included significantly low 2,3-diphosphoglycerate and glyceraldehyde-3-phosphate in the sera of PF. The sera of PV had significantly low levels of retinol but high levels of retinoic acid. Conclusion: Our study reveals metabolic alterations induced by Plasmodium spp. in human serum and would serve as a milestone in the development of novel anti-malarial strategies.

(Na J, Khan A, Kim JK, Wadood A, Choe YL, Walker DI, Jones DP, Lim CS, Park YH. Discovery of metabolic alterations in the serum of patients infected with Plasmodium spp. by high-resolution metabolomics. Metabolomics. 2019 Dec 23;16(1):9. doi: 10.1007/s11306-019-1630-2. PMID: 31872321.)

2

RETINOIDS, RACE AND THE PATHOGENESIS OF DENGUE HEMORRHAGIC FEVER

Med Hypotheses 2013 Dec;81(6):1069-74. doi: 10.1016/j.mehy.2013.08.004.
Retinoids, race and the pathogenesis of dengue hemorrhagic fever
Anthony R Mawson

Abstract

Dengue hemorrhagic fever (DHF) is the most significant mosquito-borne viral disease worldwide in terms of illness, mortality and economic cost, but the pathogenesis of DHF is not well understood and there is no specific treatment or vaccine. Based on evidence of DHF-associated liver involvement, it is proposed that dengue virus and retinoids interact to cause cholestatic liver damage; this results in the spillage of toxic amounts and concentrations of stored retinoids into the circulation, which induce the features of the disease, including severe arthralgia, bone pain, thrombocytopenia, headache, and gastrointestinal symptoms. While retinoids in low concentration are essential for numerous biological functions, they are prooxidant, cytotoxic, mutagenic and teratogenic in higher concentration, especially when unbound to protein, and an endogenous form of vitamin A intoxication is recognized in cholestasis. The model accounts for a number of hitherto unexplained observations related to dengue virus infection, e.g., 1) repeat infections are more severe than initial dengue virus infections, 2) the incidence of dengue has increased dramatically worldwide in recent decades; 3) DHF is less prevalent in people of African ancestry than among those of other racial backgrounds; and 4) infants are protected from dengue. The retinoid toxicity hypothesis of DHF predicts the co-existence of low serum concentrations of retinol coupled with high concentrations of retinoic acid and an increased percentage of retinyl esters to total vitamin A. Subject to such tests, it may be possible to treat DHF effectively using drugs that target the metabolism and expression of retinoids.

Key Words: dengue; virus; retinoids; liver; pathogenesis; cholestasis; fever; bone pain; headache; health disparities

Background

Dengue, a mosquito-borne viral infection, causes a severe flu-like illness with a potentially lethal complication – dengue hemorrhagic fever (DHF). Dengue is the most significant mosquito-borne viral disease worldwide in terms of illness, death, and economic cost, due to the lack of an approved vaccine or antiviral agents. The disease is endemic in more than 100 countries in Africa, the Americas, the Eastern Mediterranean, South-east Asia and the Western Pacific. Currently, the most seriously affected areas are South-east Asia and the Western Pacific. During epidemics of dengue, infection rates among those who have not been previously exposed to the virus can reach 80% to 90%.[1]

Infection with dengue viruses is a threat to about 2.5 billion people, and 50-100 million are infected each year. An estimated 500,000 people with DHF require hospitalization annually, a large proportion of whom are children. About 2.5% of those affected die. The spread of dengue is attributed to an expanding geographic distribution of dengue viruses and their mosquito vectors, the most important being the predominantly urban species *Aedes aegypti*. Disease prevalence has increased dramatically in recent years.

Dengue viruses are transmitted to humans through the bites of infective female *Aedes* mosquitoes, which usually acquire the virus while feeding on the blood of an infected person. Dengue fever seldom causes death and is more severe in older children and adults. DHF or dengue shock syndrome (DSS) can present with a diverse clinical spectrum. The classical incapacitating disease has an abrupt onset with a sudden rise in temperature accompanied by facial flush, hepatomegaly and, in severe cases, circulatory failure, and flu-like symptoms including headache, pain behind the eyes, severe muscle, bone and joint pains, extreme fatigue, and rash. Fever usually continues for 2-7 days and can reach 41°C, occasionally with convulsions. Characteristic features include capillary leakage with pleural and pulmonary effusions resulting from increased vascular permeability, accompanied by thrombocytopenia and leukopenia; liver damage, indicated by increases in aspartate aminotransferase and alanine aminotransferase; hypotesion, hemoconcentration and hypoalbuminemia; gastrointestinal bleeding and spontaneous bleeding from the gums and nose. In severe cases the temperature drops after a few days, followed by signs of circulatory failure, shock and death within 12-24 hours. Untreated, complicated DHF can have a 50% mortality rate. However, with appropriate treatment, recovery may be rapid.[2]

There is no specific treatment for dengue fever and no vaccine is available. Since DHF is caused by four closely related virus serotypes of the genus *Flavivirus*, a successful vaccine must immunize against all four types. At present, the pathogenesis is not well understood, and few animal models are available to test immune responses to potential vaccines.[3]

A current hypothesis is that sudden capillary leakage syndrome, the principal pathologic event in DHF/DSS, is generated by cytokines released when T cells attack dengue-infected cells.[4] Dengue shock can be accompanied by increased peripheral vascular resistance and raised diastolic blood pressure. High concentrations of interferon-α are recorded 1-2 days after the onset of fever. At the end of the febrile period, coincident with onset of vascular permeability, high concentrations of soluble interleukin-2 receptor, soluble tumor necrosis factor, soluble CD4, soluble CD8, interleukin-2, and interferon-γ are noted. DHF patients have reduced circulating nitric oxide and enhanced interleukin-10 concentrations in blood. Disease severity correlates with markers of immune activation, e.g., interleukins 6 and 8, tumor necrosis factor-α, interferons n1 and γ, soluble tumor necrosis factor-α receptor, and complement components 3a and 5a. Thrombocytopenia is almost always present in patients with dengue, with platelet nadirs as low as 5,000 cells per μL. During the recovery period, platelet numbers rise promptly. With increasing cardiovascular compromise, diastolic pressure rises towards the systolic and pulse pressure narrows. Many T cells show an apoptotic phenotype. However, the hypothesis that severe dengue disease is associated with T-cell immunopathology is inconsistent with the fact that heterologous T-cell responses are not needed to produce DHF in infants; in fact, infants from Southeast Asia do not develop clinical dengue illnesses until around 6 months of age.[4]

Liver injury associated with dengue infection has been described since the 1960s and appears to be universal in patients with DHF. In most patients, liver dysfunction is mild or moderate and presents primarily as elevation of serum aminotransferases; in others, the clinical manifestations of liver disease can include jaundice, hepatomegaly and ascites, leading to acute liver failure, encephalopathy and death.[5] Mortality risks increase in patients with severe hepatitis and encephalopathy.

In a study from South Asia on mortality in DHF, liver involvement was found to prolong the normally self-limiting clinical course of dengue infection and the prognosis was worsened by severe liver involvement.

Complications such as bleeding, renal failure, encephalopathy and cholecystitis were also more frequent in patients with severe hepatitis.[6]

Liver Involvement and the Retinoid Toxicity Hypothesis

The hypothesis proposed here is that the diverse manifestations of DHF are due to interactions between dengue virus and endogenous retinoids (vitamin A and its congeners), leading to retinoid receptor-induced activation of hepatic stellate cells and damage to the liver and the spillage of stored retinoids into the circulation in toxic concentrations. Over 80% of body stores of vitamin A are contained in the liver, and in sufficient quantity to last the average adult about two years without the need for additional intake.[7]

Retinoids are fat-soluble signaling molecules that are mainly derived from the diet as preformed vitamin A or as provitamin A carotenoids and are essential for multiple biological functions, including embryonic development, vision, gene expression, tissue differentiation, growth, immune function, and mucus secretion.[8] Retinoic acid (RA), the active form of vitamin A in most cellular systems, binds to and activates the transcription of many target genes via the retinoic acid receptors and the retinoid X receptors.[9] While retinoids in low concentrations act as growth factors, higher concentrations are prooxidant, cytotoxic, mutagenic and teratogenic, especially when unbound to protein.[10,11]

Similarities to Hypervitaminosis A There are strong parallels between the manifestations of DHF and those of hypervitaminosis A. Most if not all of the signs and symptoms of DHF have a counterpart in the manifestations of hypervitaminosis A (see Table 1, below). The manifestations of DHF include sudden fever lasting 3-7 days, intense headache (especially behind the eyes), muscle, bone and joint pain (ankles, knees and elbows), vomiting, diarrhea, abdominal pain, skin and neck flushing, rash on arms and legs, severe itching, peeling of skin and hair loss, minor bleeding (nose or gums), heavy menstrual periods, and extreme fatigue, with capillary leakage, thrombocytopenia, flu-like symptoms and convulsions.[12] These features are also seen in the retinoic acid syndrome induced by the treatment of acute promyelocytic leukemia with retinoic acid[13, 13A] and in acute hypervitaminosis A associated with supplements or excess dietary intakes of vitamin A-containing foods such as liver.

Ingestion of polar bear and seal liver by members of early Arctic expeditions led to severe illness, including loss of skin from head to foot, drowsiness, severe headache and vomiting, alopecia, enteritis, emaciation and pneumonia, due to vitamin A intoxication. In rats fed hypervitaminotic diets, softening and fracture of bones, profuse and sudden internal hemorrhage and occasional death have also been noted.[11,14]

Table 1 Similarities between the signs and symptoms of dengue hemorrhagic fever and of hypervitaminosis A Sources: Refs. [1,2,4,5, 11-18]

Signs/Symptoms	Dengue Hemorrhagic Fever	Hypervitaminosis A
High fever	+	+
Chills	+	+
Rhinitis	+	+
Headache	+	+
Arthralgia	+	+
Myalgia	+	+
Bone pain	+	+
Malaise	+	+
Fatigue	+	+
Cough	+	+
Acute respiratory distress	+	+
Peripheral edema	+	+
Thrombocytopenia	+	+
Hepatitis	+	+

Acute vitamin A poisoning is associated with fever, arthralgia and arthritis, myalgia, headache, flu-like symptoms, conjunctival congestion, lymphadenopathy, pruritus, erythematous rash, weakness, anorexia, desquamation, and altered mental status. Rarely and in more severe cases, hepatosplenomegaly, miscarriage, Guillain-Barré syndrome[15] and thrombocytopenic purpura have been recorded.[13, 13A] Reports have also been published of patients experiencing thrombotic episodes resulting in cerebral ischemia, facial paralysis, and dysarthria while on oral isotretinoin treatment for severe acne.[16] Bone pain and fatigue are well-documented symptoms of hypervitaminosis A.[17] Headache, another common symptom of DHF, is also a major feature of retinoid toxicity.[18] Retinoid toxicity is associated with high-to-normal or even low circulating retinol concentrations, and with increased fractions of retinyl esters circulating with plasma lipoproteins and not bound to retinol-binding protein (RBP). Symptoms usually disappear after withdrawal of vitamin A, except for occasional liver enlargement.[10,11,19-21]

A clue to understanding the pathogenesis of DHF may lie in observations implicating the liver in the disease. In addition to being the target of viruses that are specifically hepatotropic (e.g., hepatitis A, B, C and E), the liver is also affected by viruses that primarily target other tissues, including dengue viruses.[22] The incidence of hepatic dysfunction is greater in dengue shock syndrome (DSS) and dengue hemorrhagic fever (DHF) than in milder cases.[23] Among children with dengue infection, liver involvement varies from mild injury with elevation of transaminases to severe injury with jaundice and liver failure.[24] In studies from India and Thailand, dengue infection was found to be the most important cause of acute liver failure in children, contributing to 18.5% and 34.3% of cases, respectively.[25,26] In a recent study of 110 children ages 2 months to 14 years with serologically-positive dengue fever, the spectrum of hepatic manifestations included hepatomegaly (79%), hepatic tenderness (56%), jaundice (4.5%), raised levels of aspartate transaminase (93%), alanine transaminase (78%), alkaline phosphatase (57%), prolonged prothrombin time (20%), reduced levels of serum albumin (66%) and abnormal abdomen ultrasound (65%).[27]

Outline of the Model

1. Dengue virus infection activates the retinoid cascade in the liver, leading to increased retinoic acid production and retinoic acid receptor (RAR) activation and expression within the hepatic cell nuclei, causing inflammation and liver damage.

It is proposed that DHF-induced increased RAR activation inhibits the production and secretion of retinol binding-protein (RBP), possibly via a process of feedback inhibition,[28] which lowers serum retinol concentrations and simultaneously increases the accumulation and expression of retinoids in the liver. In the one published report on retinoids in DHF, serum retinol was reduced in acute DHF,[29] as the present model predicts. However, other retinoids, including retinyl esters and retinoic acid, have not been assessed in DHF. Increased RAR expression in the liver induces inflammation and tissue damage, consistent with the known role of excessive vitamin A in liver damage.[20] Polar retinol metabolites extracted from liver tissues of rats were found to cause marked hepatocyte damage in a concentration- and time-dependent manner, due to apoptosis, as shown by increased of sub-G1 cellular events, rapid loss of mitochondrial membrane potential, and activation of caspase-9 and -3.[30]

Kupffer cells, in addition to being the source of macrophages in the liver, play a critical role in hypervitaminosis A. Vitamin A activates Kupffer cells through INF-γ production by activated T-lymphocytes,[31] and activated Kupffer cells potentiate liver toxicity even with low levels of other hepatotoxins such as alcohol.[32] The nonparenchymal Ito (or stellate) cells contain about 90% of total liver vitamin A and are the primary source of the extracellular matrix deposition in liver fibrosis and of the apoptotic mediators involved in fibrosis.[33] During hepatic fibrosis, the normally quiescent vitamin A-storing stellate cells transform into myofibroblastic cells and lose their intracellular droplets of retinyl esters, the storage form of vitamin A. The loss of retinyl esters is associated with increased retinoic acid formation, which in turn facilitates TGF-beta-mediated liver fibrogenesis.[34] This phenotypic transformation induces potent pro-inflammatory and pro-fibrogenic activities and is underpinned by changes in the expression of numerous genes.[35]

BALB/c mice inoculated intravenously with dengue virus developed extensive damage to the liver around the central vein and portal tracts, consisting of hepatocyte injury, steatosis, swelling, necrosis, and evidence of vascular damage, including hemorrhage, which is characteristic of dengue-induced hepatitis. Hepatic lesions, first noted 2 days post-infection, were more extensive after the seventh day in association with increased alanine aminotransferase and aspartate aminotransferase levels. These changes were self-limiting, with a marked reduction of liver damage by 49 days post-infection. Virus antigens were detected in hepatocytes, Kupffer cells and vascular endothelium, suggesting virus replication in these cells that was confirmed by in situ hybridization.[36]

2. Retinoid-induced Kupffer cell activation and hepatotoxicity due to DHF infection lead to a transient form of cholestatic liver

dysfunction, in which bile regurgitates into the circulation, raising the level of all biliary substances in the blood.[37,38]

In cholestasis, vitamin A metabolites and bile acids are refluxed from the liver and stored retinyl esters leak into the circulation via damaged hepatocytes. Metabolites of retinol, retinyl acetate, retinal, retinoic acid, retinol beta-glucuronide, retinotaurine, and other unidentified vitamin A compounds are excreted in the bile[10,39] in proportion to the total liver stores of the vitamin.[40] A variety of infections and stressors are associated with transient declines in plasma retinol concentrations.[41,42] but plasma retinol concentrations tend to rebound when the inflammatory stimulus is removed.[43] The hypothesized net effect of transient cholestasis in DHF is high circulating concentrations of retinoid metabolites and retinyl esters, with low or normal concentrations of retinol and RBP. As noted, serum retinol is reduced in acute DHF.[29]

3. Retinoic acid and stored retinyl esters released into the circulation from damaged liver cells cause the manifestations of DHF via apoptosis and necrosis.

DHF-DSS result from aberrant immune responses involving antibody-dependent enhancement of infection, thrombocytopenia, and a loss of vascular integrity, culminating in hemorrhage, shock, and occasionally in death. Studies indicate that dengue virus infection results in the induction of caspase-dependent apoptosis of cells involved in dengue pathogenesis.[44] Sepsis and septic shock are proinflammatory responses associated with an increased risk of multi-organ failure and death. In cirrhosis and severe sepsis, proinflammatory cytokines are thought to contribute to worsening liver function and the development of shock, renal failure, acute lung injury or acute respiratory distress syndrome, coagulopathy, hepatic encephalopathy, hyperglycemia, defective arginine-vasopressin secretion, and adrenal insufficiency.[45,46] As noted, DHF-DSS are associated with high concentrations of interferon (INF)-γ and other cytokines (e.g., soluble IL-2 receptor, soluble TNF, soluble CD4, soluble CD8, and IL-2) at the end of the febrile period, coincident with the onset of vascular permeability, and these correlate with the severity of dengue disease. Disease severity also correlates with reduced circulating nitric oxide and with markers of immune activation, e.g., IL-6. [4] INF regulatory factor-1 (IRF-1) is an important transcription factor involved in cell growth and apoptosis, differentiation, and antiviral and antibacterial immune responses. The proposed model is supported by the observation that retinoic acid regulates INF-y-induced

IRF-1 by affecting multiple components of the INF-γ signaling pathway, from the plasma membrane to the nuclear transcription factors.[47] Retinoic acid is inversely associated with nitric oxide production in endothelial cells.[48] Capillary leakage associated with vascular fragility in dengue is also reported in the retinoic acid syndrome (RAS) and could be due to the membrane destabilizing effects of retinoids and the associated endothelial hyperpermeability.[48A]

The hypothesis that liver damage-induced DHF-DSS is associated with alterations in retinoid metabolism is supported by a study of serum and hepatic vitamin A levels in patients with cirrhosis, where serum retinyl ester concentrations were found to be significantly higher than in controls (see Table 2, below).[49] The percentage of serum retinyl esters as a fraction of total vitamin (retinol plus esters), which is an accepted indicator of vitamin A toxicity when > 10%, was 20%.[11] One of the hallmarks of DHF is elevated IL-6.[4] Hepatic steatosis is also associated with the increased production of IL-6 and other proinflammatory cytokines by hepatocytes and nonparenchymal cells, including Kupffer cells and hepatic stellate cells.[50]

Table 2 Serum vitamin A concentrations in controls and in patients with cirrhosis Source: Ref. [49]

Variable	Controls		Patients with cirrhosis		p
	Median	Range	Median	Range	
Retinol, μg/L	259	84–1138	166	46–918	<.001
Retinyl esters, μg/L	18	0–159	42	0–152	<.001
RBP, mmol/L	2.1	< 1.1–24.2	1.8	<1.1–5.8	<.001

RBP, retinol-binding protein

To summarize the model, dengue virus-induced activation of the retinoid cascade causes liver damage and the spillage of retinoic acid and unbound retinyl esters into the circulation, inducing the manifestations of DHF, potential multiorgan failure and sepsis. It is further suggested that the severity of dengue virus infection is directly associated with the extent of preexisting liver dysfunction.

Implications and Predictions

The model provisionally explains a number of observations about dengue virus infection and offers several predictions:

1) *Repeat infections are more severe than initial dengue virus infections* The prevailing view of the pathogenesis of DHF is based on the concept of "antibody-dependent enhancement" (ADE), i.e., that antibodies acquired during a primary infection increase the number of infected cells and thus the level of viremia during secondary infection. However, the severity of dengue is not limited to DSS, and many cases do not conform to the ADE concept.[51] The present model suggests that the initial illness causes hepatic stellate cell activation, steatosis and profibrotic changes in the liver which increase the severity of DHF when subsequent infections occur, associated with enhanced retinoid toxicity.
2) *The incidence of dengue has increased dramatically worldwide in recent decades.* In addition to broadening spread of the disease via *Aedes aegypti,* the increase in incidence may also be due in part to the increased global prevalence of non-alcoholic fatty liver disease (NAFLD),[52] which appears to increase susceptibility to dengue viral infection. The presence and symptom-exacerbating effect of steatosis could explain the association between DHF and higher socioeconomic status and hence dietary intake. Indeed, in a case-control study of risk factors for DHF, based on 170 cases of DHF and 1,175 controls in a dengue sero-positive population in two Brazilian cities, Figueiredo et al.[53] found significant associations between DHF and income (OR = 6.84; 95% Confidence Interval: 4.09-11.43), education (OR = 4.67; CI: 2.35-9.27), and self-reported reported diabetes (OR = 2.75; CI: 1.12-6.73).
3) *DHF, the severe form of dengue, is less prevalent in people of African ancestry than among those of other ethnic backgrounds* Morbidity and mortality associated with dengue are lower among African descendent populations than among European and Asian descendent populations.[54,55] People of African descent living in Latin America and the Caribbean are often asymptomatic or display only mild or moderate symptoms of dengue in contrast to the more severe symptoms shown by other ethnic populations. The current explanation is that lower dengue morbidity and mortality result from innate genetic resistance.[54,55] It is of interest that people of African descent are also at reduced risk of death from yellow fever viral infection,[56-58] which similarly targets the liver and has many parallels

to DHF. Figueiredo et al,[53] in their matched case-control study in Brazil, found a significant association between DHF and white ethnicity (OR = 4.70; CI: 2.17-10.20). However, black individuals who reported being treated for hypertension had a 13-fold higher risk of DHF than those reporting no hypertension.

These observations may reflect differences in liver function, retinoid storage and metabolism in people of African descent compared to other ethnicities, due to genetic adaptations over millennia to parasitic diseases and, in particular, malaria and its effects on host vitamin A. It is known that African Americans have less intraperitoneal and liver fat and more lower extremity fat than Causasians or Hispanics, which could explain the reduced risk of African Americans for the development and progression of nonalcoholic fatty liver disease. [59] It is also known that malaria parasites selectively absorb vitamin A from the host;[60] that low vitamin A reserves are associated with increased mortality risks from malaria whereas high reserves are associated with less severe disease and reduced risks of mortality; and losses of vitamin A can lead to sickness or death from other infections.[61] The author has recently suggested that malaria parasites emerging from the liver as merozoites use their accumulated vitamin A as a membrane destabilizer to invade the red blood cells, and proposed that the characteristic features of hemolysis and anemia and other symptoms of malaria are manifestations of an endogenous form of vitamin A intoxication caused by the parasites, associated with high concentrations of RA.[62]

These considerations suggest that among sub-Saharan Africans, co-existence with malaria parasites over millennia may have created evolutionary-adaptive pressures, first, to conserve and prevent vitamin A deficiency by reducing the hepatic metabolism of vitamin A; and secondly, to reduce the severity of malaria symptoms by lowering vitamin A stores in the liver and sequestering it in the lower extremities, thereby reducing parasite ingestion of the vitamin. These adaptations could explain why dengue and yellow fever are less harmful to people of African descent than those of other racial/ethnic groups.

In sum, exposure to malaria parasites may have led to a tendency among sub-Saharan Africans in their ancestral geographic and nutritional environment to accumulate less vitamin A and to store it more efficiently in the liver than inhabitants of areas of lesser exposure, thereby rendering them less prone to DHF, and to death from yellow fever. However, with adoption of western-style dietary patterns, Africans and people of other ethnicities who develop fatty liver and associated features of the metabolic syndrome, including hypertension and diabetes, could be at increased risk of DHF. Indeed, significant risk factors for DHF include diabetes mellitus, hypertension and obesity, all of which are associated with nonalcoholic steatohepatitis.[53,63] Indeed, the postulated state of reduced vitamin A metabolism could render people of African descent particularly sensitive to the toxic effects of vitamin A. This could explain the dramatically higher rate of colorectal cancer among African Americans compared to native Africans (60/100,000 compared to < 1/100,000), the latter of whom consume less protein, fat, meat, saturated fat, cholesterol and vitamin A than the former.[64]

4) *Infants are protected from dengue.* Infants do not develop clinical symptoms of dengue until the age of 6 months.[4] The present model suggests that infants are protected from dengue due to low hepatic reserves of vitamin A. In fact, infants up to 6 months of age have very low liver stores of the vitamin.[65] In one study, liver samples taken at autopsy from 170 American children ages 0-15 years showed that the median liver vitamin A concentration at birth was low (11 μg retinol/g) and remained constant to 3 months, then increased rapidly to 4 years (130 μg/g) and remained constant into adolescence. Among infants less than 3 months of age, liver vitamin A concentrations ≤ 20 μg/g were present in about two-thirds, whereas virtually all infants ≥ 6 months showed an adequate vitamin A status, defined as liver stores > 20 μg retinol/g liver.[66] Reduced risks of DHF among infants under 6 months of age could therefore be due to low liver stores of vitamin A and hence to a lessened risk of virus-associated hepatocyte inflammation and injury.

Conclusions

Is it proposed that DHF-DSS result from interactions between dengue viruses and retinoids in the liver, triggering viral replication and disease pathogenesis, and that disease manifestations (e.g., fever, severe arthralgia, bone pain, thrombocytopenia, headache, and gastrointestinal symptoms) are caused by the damaging effects of dengue virus-induced activation of hepatocytes and the resulting spillage of toxic retinoids (i.e., retinyl esters and retinoic acid) into the circulation.

The model accounts for a number of hitherto unexplained observations related to dengue virus infection, e.g., 1) repeat infections are more severe than initial dengue virus infections, 2) the incidence of dengue has increased dramatically worldwide in recent decades; 3) DHF is less prevalent in people of African ancestry than among those of other racial backgrounds; and 4) infants are protected from dengue. The model could be tested by comparing retinoid profiles in patients with DHF and uninfected controls. Subject to positive outcomes of such tests, the model suggests that DHF could be treated effectively using drugs that target the metabolism and expression of retinoids and/or by procedures that reduce their concentration.

References

1. Simmons CP, Farrar JJ, Chau NVV, Wills B. Dengue. NEJM 2013; 366(15):1-10.
2. Raheel U, Faheem M, Riaz MN, Kanwal N, Javed F, Zaidi Nu, Qadri I. Dengue fever in the Indian Subcontinent: an overview. J Infect Dev Ctries 2011; 5(4):239-47.
3. World Health Organization. Dengue and dengue hemorrhagic fever. Fact sheet N°117. Geneva: World Health Organization; May 2008. Available from: http://www.who.int/mediacentre/factsheets/fs117/en/
4. Halstead S. Dengue. Lancet 2007; 370: 1644-1652.
5. Chhinaa RS, Goyala O, Chhinaa DK, Goyala P, Kumar R, Purim S. Liver function tests in patients with dengue viral infection. Dengue Bulletin 2008; 32:110-117.
6. Parkash O, Almas A, Jafri SMW, Hamid S, Akhtar J, Alishah H. Severity of acute hepatitis and its outcome in patients with dengue fever in a tertiary care hospital Karachi, Pakistan (South Asia). BMC Gastroenterology 2010, 10:43 http://www.biomedcentral.com/1471-230X/10/43
7. De Luca LM, Creek KE. Vitamin A and the liver. Prog Liver Dis 1986; 8:81-98.
8. Litwak G (Ed.) Vitamin A: Vitamins and Hormones, Vol. 75. San Diego, CA: Elsevier Academic Press, 2007.
9. Lane MA, Bailey SJ. Role of retinoid signalling in the adult brain. Prog Neurobiol 2005; 75:275-93.
10. Olson JA. Vitamin A—functions, dietary requirements and safety in humans. In: Ziegler EE, Filer LJ Jr, editors. Present knowledge in nutrition. 7th ed. Washington, DC: International Life Sciences Institute Press, 2001; pp. 109-19.
11. Penniston KL, Tanumihardjo SA. The acute and chronic toxic effects of vitamin A. Am J Clin Nutr 2006; 83:191-201.
http://www.health.qld.gov.au/dengue/dengue_fever/disease.asp

12. Patatanian E, Thompson DF. Retinoic acid syndrome: a review. J Clin Pharmacol Ther 2008; 33:331-338.
13. A. Estival JL, Dupin M, Kanstakis J, Combemale P. Capillary leak syndrome induced by Acitretin. Br J Dermatol 2004; 150(1):150-2.
14. Rodahl K, Moore T. The vitamin A content and toxicity of bear and seal liver. Biochem J 1943; 37:166-168. http://www.biochemj.org/bj/037/0166/0370166.pdf
15. Pritchard J. Guillain Barré in 13-cis-retinoic acid. Br Med J 2004; 328:1537.
16. Laroche ML, Macian-Montoro F, Merle L, Vallat JM. Cerebral ischemia probably related to isotretinoin. Ann Pharmacother 2007; 41:1073-6.
17. Binkley N, Brueger D. Hypervitaminosis A and bone. Nutr Rev 2000; 58:138-144.
18. Aboulafia DM, Norris D, Henry D, Grossman RJ, Thommes J, Bundow D, Yocum RC, Stevens V. 9-cis-retinoic acid capsules in the treatment of AIDS-related Kaposi sarcoma: results of a phase 2 multicenter clinical trial. Arch Dermatol 2003; 139:178-86.
19. Moore T. Vitamin A. New York: Elsevier North Holland, Inc., 1957.
20. Leo MA, Lieber CS. New pathway of retinol metabolism in liver microsomes. J Biol Chem 1985; 260:5228-31.
21. Johnson-Davis KL, Moore SJ, Owen WE, et al. A rapid HPLC method used to establish pediatric reference intervals for vitamins A and E. Clin Chim Acta 2009; 405:35-8.
22. Adams DH, Hubscher SG. Systemic viral infections and collateral damage in the liver. Am J Pathol 2006; 168(4):1057-1059.
23. Seneviratne SL, Malavige GN, de Silva HJ. Pathogenesis of liver involvement during dengue viral infections. Trans Roy Soc Trop Med Hyg 2006; 100(7):608–14.
24. Petdachai W. Hepatic dysfunction in children with dengue shock syndrome. Dengue Bull 2005; 29:112–7.
25. Kumar R, Tripathi P, Tripathi S, Kanodia A, Venkatesh V. Prevalence of dengue infection in north Indian children with acute hepatic failure. Ann Hepatol 2008; 7(1):59–62.
26. Poovorawan Y, Hutagalung Y, Chongsrisawat V, Boudville I, Bock HL. Dengue virus infection: a major cause of acute hepatic failure in Thai children. Ann Trop Paediatr 2006; 26(1):17–23.
27. Jagadishkumar K, Jain P, Manjunath VG, Umesh L. Hepatic involvement in dengue fever in children. Iran J Pediatr 2012; 22(2):231-6.

28. Barua AB, Duitsman PK, Kostic D, Barua M, Olson JA. Reduction of serum retinol levels following a single oral dose of all-trans retinoic acid in humans. Int J Vitam Nutr Res 1997; 67:423-6.
29. Klassen P, Biesalski HK, Mazariegos M, Solomons NW, Fürst P. Classic dengue fever affects levels of circulating antioxidants. Nutrition 2004; 20(6):542-7.
30. Dan Z, Popov Y, Patsenker E, Preimel D, Liu C, Wang XD, Seitz HK, Schuppan D, Stickel F. Hepatotoxicity of alcohol-induced polar retinol metabolites involves apoptosis via loss of mitochondrial membrane potential. FASEB J 2005; 19(7):845-7.
31. Sim W, Abril E, Earnest D. Mechanisms of Kupffer cell activation in hypervitaminosis A. In Wisse E, Knook D, Decker K (eds). Cells of the hepatic sinusoid. The Kupffer Cell Foundation, Riiswijk, 1989: 91-93.
32. Mobley SA, Sim W, Sipes IG. Repeated exposure to subclinical doses of hepatotoxicant enhances liver injury with hypervitaminosis A: a possible cause for chronic liver disease. Gastroenterology 1989; 96:A689.
33. Li D, Friedman SL. Liver fibrogenesis and the role of hepatic stellate cells: new insights and prospects for therapy. J Gastroenterol Hepatol 1999; 17:618-33.
34. Okuno M, Kojima S, Akita K, Matsushima-Nishiwaki R, Adachi S, Sano T, Takano Y, Takai K, Obora A, Yasuda I, Shiratori Y, Okano Y, Shimada J, Suzuki Y, Muto Y, Moriwaki Y. Retinoids in liver fibrosis and cancer. Front Biosci 2002; 7:d204-18.
35. Mann J, Mann DA. Transcriptional regulation of hepatic stellate cells. Adv Drug Deliv Rev 2009; 61(7-8):497-512.
36. Paes MV, Lenzi HL, Nogueira AC, Nuovo GJ, Pinhão AT, Mota EM, Basílio-de-Oliveira CA, Schatzmayr H, Barth OM, Alves AM. Hepatic damage associated with dengue-2 virus replication in liver cells of BALB/c mice. Lab Invest 2009; 89(10):1140-51.
37. Popper H, Schaffner F. Cholestasis. Chapter 148 in Berk JE (ed.), Gastroenterology, Vol 5, Fourth edition. W.B. Saunders Co: Philadeplphia, 1985:2697-2731.
38. Ramanthan V, Hensley G, French S, Eysselein V, Chung D, Reicher S, Pham B. Hypervitaminosis A inducing intra-hepatic cholestasis—a rare case report. Exp Mol Pathol 2010; 898:324-325.
39. Frolik CA. Metabolism of retinoids. In Sporn MB, Roberts AB, Goodman DS (eds.), The Retinoids. New York: Academic Press, 1984, pp. 177-208.
40. Hicks VA, Gunning DB, Olson JA. Metabolism, plasma transport and biliary excretion of radioactive vitamin A and its metabolites as a

function of liver reserves of vitamin A in the rat. J Nutr 1984; 114(7):1327-33.
41. Mitra AK, Alvarez MA, Wahed MA, Fuchs GJ, Stephenson CB. Predictors of serum retinol in children with shigellosis. Am J Clin Nutr 1998; 68:1088-1094.
42. Schweigert FJ. Inflammation–induced changes in the nutritional biomarkers serum retinol and carotenoids. Curr Opin Clin Nutr Metab Care 2001; 4:477-481.
43. Gieng SH, Green MH, Green JB, Rosales FJ. Model-based compartmental analysis indicates a reduced mobilization of hepatic vitamin A during inflammation in rats. J Lipid Res 2007; 48:904-913.
44. Brown MG, Huang YY, Marshall JS, King CA, Hoskin DW, Anderson R. Dramatic caspase-dependent apoptosis in antibody-enhanced dengue virus infection of human mast cells *J Leuk Biol* 2009; 85:71-80.
45. Gustot T, Durand F, Lebrec D, Vincent JL, Moreau R. Severe sepsis in cirrhosis. Hepatology 2009; 50(6):2022-33.
46. Clark IA, Alleva LM, Vissel B. The roles of TNF in brain dysfunction and disease. Pharmacol Ther 2010; 128(3):519-48.
47. Luo XM, Ross AC. Physiological and receptor-selective retinoids modulate Interferon γ signaling by increasing the expression, nuclear localization, and functional activity of interferon regulatory factor-1. J Biol Chem 2005; 280:36228-36236.
48. Cho DH, Choy YJ, Jo SA, Nam JH, Jung SC, Jo I. Retinoic acid decreases nitric oxide production in endothelial cells: a role of phosphorylation of endothelial nitric oxide synthase at Ser^{1179} . Biochem Biophys Res Commun 2005; 326(4):703-710.
48A. Miyoshi T, Arai T, Yamashita K, Sasada M, Uchiyama T. NB4 cells treated with all-trans retinoic acid generate toxic reactive oxygen species that cause endothelial hyperpermeability. Leuk Res 2010; 34(3):373-8. doi: 10.1016/j.leukres.2009.05.022.
49. Ukleja A, Scolapio JS, McConnell JP, Spivey JR, Dickson RC, Nguyen JH, O'Brien PC. Nutritional assessment of serum and hepatic vitamin A levels in patients with cirrhosis. J Parenter Enteral Nutr 2002; 26(3):184-8.
50. Stefan N, Kantartziz K, Häring HU. Causes and metabolic consequences of fatty liver. Endocr Rev 2008; 29:939-960.
51. Deparis X, Maréchal V, Matheus S. Pathophysiological mechanisms of dengue fever: critical review of current concepts. Med Trop (Mars) 2009; 69(4):351-7.
52. Lazo M, Clark JM. The epidemiology of nonalcoholic fatty liver disease: a global perspective. Semin Liver Dis 2008; 28(4):339-350.

53. Figueiredo MA, Rodrigues LC, Barreto ML, Lima JW, Costa MC, Morato V, Blanton R, Vasconcelos PF, Nunes MR, Teixeira MG. Allergies and diabetes as risk factors for dengue hemorrhagic fever: results of a case control study. PLoS Negl Trop Dis 2010; 4(6):e699.
54. Halstead SB, Streit TG, Lafontant J, Putvatana R, Russel K, Sun W, Thasan N, Hayes C, Watts D. Haiti: absence of dengue hemorrhagic fever despite hyperendemic dengue virus transmission. Am J Trop Med 2001; 65(3):180-183.
55. Sierra B, Kouri G, Guzman MG. Race: a risk factor for dengue hemorrhagic fever. Arch Virol 2007; 52:533-543.
56. Kiple K, King V. Another dimension to the black diaspora: diet, disease and racism. Cambridge: Cambridge University Press, 1981.
57. Quaresma JA, Barros VL, Pagliari C, Fernandes ER, Guedes F, Takakura CF, Andrade HF Jr, Vasconcelos PF, Duarte MI. Revisiting the liver in human yellow fever: virus-induced apoptosis in hepatocytes associated with TGF-beta, TNF-alpha and NK cells activity. Virology 2006; 345(1):22-30.
58. Rowland M, Plackett TP, Smith R. Yellow fever vaccine-associated viscerotropic disease. Milit Med 2012; 177:467-469.
59. Guerrero R, Vega GL, Grundy SM, Browning JD. Ethnic differences in hepatic steatosis: an insulin resistance paradox? Hepatology 2009; 49(3):791-801. doi: 10.1002/hep.22726.59.
60. Mizuno Y, Kawazu SI, Kano S, Watanabe N, Matsuura T, Ohtomo H. In-vitro uptake of vitamin A by Plasmodium falciparum. Ann Trop Med Parasitol 2003; 97(3):237-43.
61. Friedman JF, Kurtis JD, Mtalib R, Opollo M, Lanar DE, Duffy PE. Malaria is related to decreased nutritional status among male adolescents and adults in the setting of intense perennial transmission. J Infect Dis 2003; 188(3):449-57.
62. Mawson AR. The pathogenesis of malaria: a new perspective. Pathogens and Global Health 2013; 107(3):122-129.
63. Lee MS, Hwang KP, Chen TC, Lu PL, Chen TP. Clinical characteristics of dengue and dengue hemorrhagic fever in a medical center of southern Taiwan during the 2002 epidemic. J Microbiol Immunol Infect 2006; 39(2):121-9.
64. O'Keefe SJ, Chung D, Mahmoud N, Sepulveda AR, Manafe M, Arch J, Adada H, van der Merwe T. Why do African Americans get more colon cancer than Native Africans? J Nutr 2007; 137(1 Suppl):175S-182S.
65. Mactier H, Weaver LT. Vitamin A and preterm infants: what we know, what we don't know, and what we need to know. Arch Dis Child Fetal Neonatal Ed 2005; 90:F103-F108.

66. Olson JA, Gunning DB, Tilton RA. Liver concentrations of vitamin A and carotenoids, as a function of age and other parameters, of American children who died of various causes. Am J Clin Nutr 1984; 39:903-910.

3

MALARIA, EPSTEIN-BARR VIRUS INFECTION, AND THE PATHOGENESIS OF BURKITT'S LYMPHOMA

Int J Cancer 2017 Nov 1;141(9):1849-1855. doi: 10.1002/ijc.30885
Malaria, Epstein-Barr virus infection and the pathogenesis of Burkitt's lymphoma
Anthony R Mawson, Suvankar Majumdar
PMID: 28707393 DOI: 10.1002/ijc.30885
https://pubmed.ncbi.nlm.nih.gov/28707393/

Abstract

A geographical and causal connection has long been recognized between malaria, Epstein-Barr virus (EBV) infection and Burkitt's lymphoma (BL), but the underlying mechanisms remain obscure. Potential clues are that the malaria parasite *Plasmodium falciparum* selectively absorbs vitamin A from the host and depends on it for its biological activities; secondly, alterations in vitamin A (retinoid) metabolism have been implicated in many forms of cancer, including BL. The first author has proposed that the merozoite-stage malaria parasite, emerging from the liver, uses its absorbed vitamin A as a cell membrane destabilizer to invade the red blood cells, causing anemia and other signs and symptoms of the disease as manifestations of an endogenous form of hypervitaminosis A (Mawson AR. Path Global Health 2013; 107(3):122-129). Repeated episodes of malaria would therefore be expected to expose the tissues of affected individuals to potentially toxic doses of vitamin A. It is proposed that such episodes activate latent EBV infection, which in turn activates retinoid-responsive genes. Expression of these genes enhances viral replication and induces germinal center (GC) B cell expansion, activation-induced cytidine deaminase (AID) expression, and c-myc translocation, which in turn predisposes to BL. Thus, an endogenous form of retinoid toxicity related to malaria infection may be the common factor linking frequent malaria, EBV infection and BL, whereby prolonged exposure of lymphatic tissues to high concentrations of retinoids may combine to induce B-cell translocation and increase the risk of Burkitt's lymphoma.

What's New?

The malaria parasite *Plasmodium falciparum* selectively absorbs vitamin A from the host and is hypothesized to use it as a cell membrane destabilizer to invade the red blood cells, contributing thereby to the signs and symptoms of the disease. Repeated episodes of malaria would therefore be expected to expose the tissues of affected individuals to periodic bursts of potentially toxic doses of vitamin A, particularly fatty tissues such as the brain and lymphatics. It is proposed that such episodes activate latent EBV infection and in turn activate retinoid-responsive genes; furthermore, expression of these genes enhances viral replication and induces germinal center (GC) B cell expansion, activation-induced cytidine deaminase (AID) expression, and c-myc translocation, which predisposes to BL.

Introduction

Burkitt's lymphoma (BL) is a cancer of the lymphatic system named after Denis Burkitt, an Irish surgeon who first described the disease while working in equatorial Africa.[1] BL is an aggressive, high-grade malignancy of the antibody-producing B lymphocytes and occurs most frequently in children ages 4-7 years in areas with endemic malaria.[2] The genes for making antibodies (immunoglobulins) are located on chromosomes 14, 2 and 22, and are expressed only in B lymphocytes. In over 80% of the cases of BL there is a reciprocal chromosomal translocation between chromosomes 8 and 14, designated t(8;14). Chromosomal translocations involve non-homologous joining of the ends of DNA breaks that occur in at least two different places in the genome simultaneously. The breakpoint in chromosome 8 coincides with the location of a proto-oncogene (*c-myc* on band q24), while the breakpoint on the other partner chromosome is an immunoglobulin chain locus.[3,4] The translocation of c-myc near to an Ig locus leads to deregulation and constitutive expression of *c-myc*, the overall effect being uncontrolled proliferation and a reduced threshold for the induction of apoptosis.[5] MYC was first discovered in a patient with BL and is one of the most commonly activated genes in human cancers. Classified as a Non-Hodgkin's lymphoma (NHL), BL has the fastest doubling time among human tumors.

Burkitt noted that the geographic distribution of BL corresponds closely to that of malaria, especially the most severe form induced by *Plasmodium falciparum*, a protozoan parasite transmitted by the female Anopheles mosquito. Malaria infections profoundly affect the B cell compartment, inducing polyclonal activation and hypersecretion of antibodies, resulting in hyper-gammaglobulinemia.[6,7] These observations suggested an infectious link between exposure to malaria and subsequent BL and led to the discovery of the first human oncogenic virus, Epstein-Barr virus.[8]

A herpesvirus, EBV is a potent transforming virus for human B cells that has been implicated in the pathogenesis of numerous malignancies.[9] In developing countries, EBV is typically acquired in early childhood, with no specific clinical features. In developed countries the infection is generally delayed until adolescence and is associated with infectious mononucleosis ("glandular fever"). Worldwide, over 90% of people are infected with EBV during their lifetime.[10] After infection, EBV persists in a latent state throughout life, selectively targeting memory B lymphocytes. Immunodeficiencies resulting from diseases such as HIV or malaria can lead to the reactivation and outgrowth of EBV-infected cells.[11]

Three clinically distinct variants of BL are recognized: endemic, sporadic, and HIV-associated forms. *Endemic BL* occurs in geographic regions where malaria is common and is the most frequent type of tumor in African children, accounting for 30-50% of all childhood cancer in equatorial Africa, with an estimated incidence of 3-6 cases per 100,000 children per year.[12] Endemic BL often presents with jaw swelling, the most frequent site of tumor involvement, and is highly age-dependent, occurring primarily in young children. Over 90% of cases are positive for EBV. In parts of sub-Saharan Africa where access to necessary medication remains limited, BL often proves fatal. The illness and associated deformities cause great suffering; tumors develop in the lymph nodes, causing the tongue to swell and cheeks to bulge, making it increasingly difficult for patients to eat. *Sporadic BL* often presents with abdominal tumors that give rise to abdominal pain or swelling, and only 10-15% of sporadic cases are EBV-positive. *HIV-associated BL* is an AIDS-defining malignancy in which about one-third of cases are EBV-positive.[13]

Persons with endemic EBV have a higher prevalence of *P. falciparum* malaria and a higher *P. falciparum* genetic diversity score than controls,[14] but the relative roles of the malaria parasite and EBV in the development of BL remain unclear. One theory is that *P. falciparum* malaria-induced polyclonal B-cell expansion and EBV reactivation increase the likelihood of a *c-myc* oncogene translocation, and hence the development of BL; another theory is that malaria infection impairs EBV-specific T-cell immunity, leading to reactivation of EBV in infected B cells and the loss of viral control.[15] Suppression of T-cell activity is suggested by the fact that children 4-9 years of age in areas endemic for malaria – the peak age-range for developing endemic BL – display inferior IFN-γ responses compared to children in areas less prone to malaria.[16]

Malaria, EBV and BL—Recent findings

The link between malaria and BL has recently been clarified by the discovery that *P. falciparum* induces expression of the gene for activation-induced cytidine deaminase (AID),[17] an enzyme that is mainly expressed in germinal center (GC) B cells and plays a pivotal role in both immunoglobulin class switch recombination and somatic hypermutation for antibody maturation. These two genetic processes result in the antibodies that protect against numerous pathogens. On the other hand, aberrant expression of AID can be a risk factor for cell leukemias and lymphomas, including the *c-myc* translocation characteristic of BL.[18,19]

In a study using a sample of tonsils obtained from individuals clinically infected with *P. falciparum* malaria and uninfected controls, Torgbor et al.[20] showed that the infected group of tonsils had high numbers of cells expressing AID and extremely high numbers of GC B cells latently infected with EBV. Extracts from *P. falciparum* infected red blood cells (RBCs) caused a strong activation of AID in tonsil B cells in vitro that appeared due in part to hemozoin, the metabolic product of hemoglobin digestion by *P. falciparum.* However, the underlying mechanism of AID activation was unclear, as was the question of why BL is specifically linked only with *P. falciparum* and not with other *Plasmodium* species, and why children are at particularly high risk of BL. The investigators concluded that *P. falciparum* infection increased two major risk factors for BL: first, the induction of AID in GC B cells; secondly, the increased frequency of EBV-infected cells in the GC, increasing the likelihood of the *c-myc* translocation. Hemozoin, however, was not as effective in inducing AID as complete extracts from *P. falciparum* infected RBCs, suggesting a role for other components of the extracts.

A second study, based on the prediction that *P. chabaudi* would lead to AID-dependent DNA damage and translocation in the GC, ultimately producing lymphoma, was carried out in a mouse model of malaria. Mice repeatedly infected with *P. chabaudi* developed prolonged expansion of GCs in which the B cells underwent rapid expansion and expressed AID. However, this did not alter the incidence of cancers arising in B cells in mice that carried a homozygous deletion of p53, thus confirming that the species of Plasmodium is important in the etiology of BL.[21]

In summary, these studies appear to provide the missing link between infection with *P. falciparum* malaria and the development of endemic BL. In the first paper, Torgbor et al.[20] showed that the human pathogen actually induces AID expression in the disease setting, but the link between this induction of AID and the DNA damage leading to lymphoma remained unclear. Subsequently, Robbiani and colleagues[21] extended this to show, in a mouse model, that AID induced by malaria was indeed a risk factor for DNA damage and lymphoma, and speculated that this mechanism occurred in and was directly related to BL.[17]

Further Clues to Understanding the Role of Malaria in Burkitt's Lymphoma

A further potential clue to understanding the roles of malaria and EBV in Burkitt's lymphoma is the observation that *P. falciparum* parasites selectively absorb vitamin A from the host in a parasitemia-dependent manner, and absorption increases with parasite maturation.[22] The parasite also appears to depend on vitamin A for its biological functions.[23] Furthermore, alterations in vitamin A metabolism have been implicated in the pathogenesis of many forms of cancer.[24]

Retinoids (the collective name for vitamin A and its congeners) are fat-soluble molecules that are essential in low concentration for numerous biological functions, including embryogenesis, normal development and tissue differentiation, but in higher concentration can be pro-oxidant, cytotoxic, apoptotic, mutagenic and teratogenic.[25] About 80% of vitamin A in the body is stored in the liver in potentially toxic concentrations. Retinyl esters are metabolized in the liver to retinol (vitamin A alcohol) and transported to the target tissues as retinol-binding protein (RBP), where it is enzymatically converted to retinaldehyde and subsequently to retinoic acid (RA), the main biologically active metabolite of vitamin A. The latter serves as a ligand for the Retinoic Acid Receptors (RARs) and the Retinoid X Receptors (RXRs), each of which has three isoforms—α, β and γ. These receptors form heterodimers and are responsible for the expression of numerous genes.[26] Retinoid toxicity is associated with high-to-normal or even low circulating retinol concentrations and with increased fractions of retinyl esters (>10% of total vitamin A) circulating with plasma lipoproteins and not bound to RBP.[27,28] Vitamin A toxicity is usually considered a relatively rare condition resulting from excessive consumption of vitamin A-containing foods, vitamin A supplementation, or from treatment with synthetic retinoids. However, retinoid intoxication can also occur endogenously, due to the sudden redistribution of liver stores of vitamin A to other tissues, e.g., when vitamin A metabolites are refluxed into the circulation in bile acids during cholestasis.[29] Due to their lipophilic and membrane-seeking properties, retinoids that are not protein-bound or properly chaperoned can inhibit cell growth and interact directly with membranes to increase their permeability and fluidity, causing hemolysis of erythrocytes and increased secretion of enzymes from lysosomes.[30]

Following their emergence from the liver, the merozoite-stage parasites invade and multiply inside RBCs, at which point the disease becomes symptomatic. Since the malaria parasite selectively absorbs vitamin A from the host and emerges from the liver presumably laden with the vitamin in high concentration, the hypothesis has been proposed[31] that the accumulated vitamin A is used by the parasites as a cell membrane destabilizer to invade the red blood cells (RBCs), causing anemia, a known manifestation of hypervitaminosis A.[32] Other signs and symptoms of malaria are likewise hypothesized to reflect vitamin A toxicity due to the widespread distribution and release of vitamin A from damaged RBCs throughout the body.

The total number of infected RBCs in a person with malaria can exceed 10 trillion (40%) out of a total of 25 trillion in the human body. Given their known lipophilicity, retinoids would be taken up by fat-storing tissues such as brain, lungs, bone marrow, and lymphatics, putatively causing the malarial symptoms of fever, chills, headache, sweats, fatigue, nausea, vomiting, and arthralgia. Persons experiencing multiple episodes of malaria may therefore be exposed to repeated toxic doses of retinoic acid delivered by merozoite-stage *P. falciparum* emerging from the liver and entering the RBCs.

Hypothesis

It is proposed that frequent and prolonged exposure of the tissues to high concentrations of retinoids resulting from *P. falciparum* infection (particularly fatty tissues such as the brain and lymphatics) increases the risk of BL as follows. Retinoids selectively absorbed from the host are used by the parasite to enter the red blood cells, putatively resulting in the signs and symptoms of malaria. This serves to activate latent EBV infection, which activates retinoic acid-responsive genes and in turn enhances EBV replication, resulting in GC B cell expansion, AID expression and *c-myc* translocation, thereby predisposing the infected individual to BL. On this hypothesis, exposure of the host tissues to periodic bursts of retinoids associated with frequent bouts of malaria induces EBV infection and enhances EBV replication; and these factors combine synergistically to increase the risk of BL via AID expression and *c-myc* translocation (see Figure 1). Since EBV infection is associated not only with increased risk of BL but also of nasopharyngeal carcinoma, acute lymphatic leukemia, and non-Burkitt's/non-Hodgkins lymphoma,[33] frequent malaria infection may provide the pathophysiological basis for the development of these other types of tumors in addition to BL.

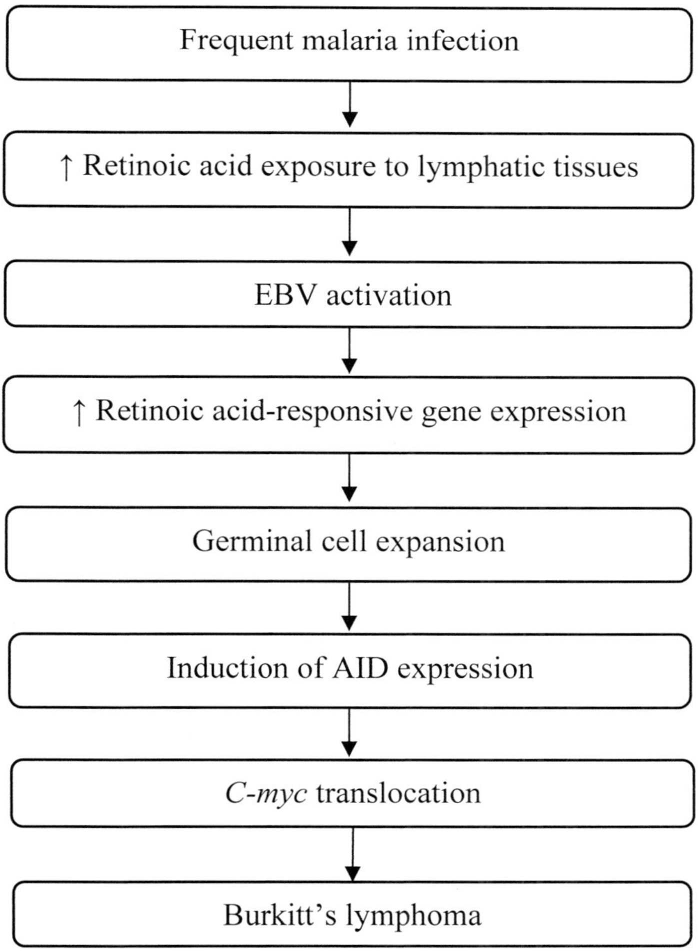

Figure 1. Retinoid toxicity model of the association between malaria, Epstein-Barr virus infection, and Burkitt's lymphoma

Uses of Retinoids in Cancer Treatment

Synthetic forms or analogs of retinoic acid (e.g., 13-cis-retinoic acid) have long been used to treat numerous forms of cancer, based on the early observation that the keratinized epithelial cells in lung cancer tissue were similar to those seen in vitamin A deficiency.[34] Indeed, retinoic acid has become the standard treatment for acute promyelocytic leukemia. Although complete remission rates have improved,[35] supplementary vitamin A using retinyl esters or synthetic retinoids have mostly temporary benefits in cancer treatment and are outweighed over time by toxic effects, e.g., the occasionally fatal "retinoic acid syndrome".[36-38] The consistent result of several long-term clinical trials of supplementary β-carotene and vitamin A for lung cancer prevention was also that these agents had no beneficial effect in cancer prevention and were associated with significant increases in lung cancer, cardiovascular disease and total mortality, notably in smokers.[39-41]

Although the current paradigm relating retinoids to carcinogenesis assumes that many cancers are associated with vitamin A deficiency,[42] growing evidence suggests that retinoid overexpression also contributes to carcinogenesis and related adverse effects, including mitochrondrial dysfunction, redox impairment, altered cell signaling, and apoptotic cell death.[25] Retinoids in pharmacological amounts and concentrations are pro-oxidant toxins that can lead to impaired brain and lung function, induce cell damage, proto-oncogene activity, proliferation and neoplastic transformation.[43-44] Dietary retinoic acid supplementation stimulates intestinal tumor formation and growth in mice.[45] Genetically engineered mouse models of colorectal cancer have provided evidence that several bioactive food components increase risk, one of which is all-trans retinoic acid.[46] Vitamin A supplementation, even at low doses, also increases the risk of all-cause mortality.[4]

Retinoic Acid and EBV

Retinoic acid plays an essential role in the differentiation of epithelial cells and participates in the regulation of several viruses.[48] For instance, treatment of undifferentiated human embryonal carcinoma cells with retinoic acid enhances susceptibility to cytomegalovirus (CMV) infection.[49] EBV can infect cells in either a latent or lytic form, and the lytic form of EBV replication is closely linked to epithelial cell differentiation. The short-chain dehydrogenase/reductase (SDR) family member 9 (*DHRS9*) cellular gene encodes alcohol dehydrogenase, a retinol-metabolizing enzyme that converts retinol to retinal and is expressed in many ciliated epithelial cell types. The switch from latent to lytic EBV is mediated by two viral immediate-early (IE) protein transcription factors, BZLF1 and BRLF1. Jones et al.[50] showed that lytic EBV infection strongly induces the transcription of *DHRS9*, an effect mediated by the BZLF1 IE protein, which binds directly to a site in the *DHRS9* promoter. BZLF1 strongly enhanced the ability of retinol to activate the RA-dependent cellular gene *CYP26A1*. These findings suggested that EBV hijacks the retinol metabolizing machinery to promote cellular differentiation and thereby enhance viral replication. Thus an EBV lytic protein (BZLF1) can enhance expression of *DHRS9* and increase the ability of retinol to activate RA-responsive cellular genes. It was suggested that this ability of EBV to stimulate retinoic acid production may help the virus to promote its own replication.

Retinoic Acid and *c-myc*

Retinoic acid is essential for the development and functions of the hematopoietic and immune systems.[51] B cells contribute to antibody production as part of the immune regulatory system and are critical for successful vaccination. Retinoic acid (RA) is an important factor in B cell maturation, proliferation, the regulation of transcription factors associated with B cell differentiation and antibody response generation. RA also augments the formation of germinal centers (GC), leading to increased primary and secondary antibody responses.[52] As B cells engage in the immune response, they express the enzyme known as activation-induced cytidine deaminase (AID), initiating the hypermutation and recombination of immunoglobulin genes, which are crucial processes for the efficient recognition and disposal of pathogens.

As noted, chromosomal translocations involving cellular myc are a hallmark of BL and central to the genetic basis of cancer.[53] This translocation may be mediated by deregulated expression of AID, which is highly expressed in GC B cells. The most common variant of *c-myc*, accounting for about 85% of cases, is t(8;14)(q24;q32).[54] Elevated activity of *c-myc* strongly stimulates cell proliferation, apoptosis, senescence, cell competition and cell differentiation.

AID creates mutations in DNA by deamination of cytosine (C) base, which converts it to uracil (U); that is, it changes a C:G (guanine) base pair into a U:G mismatch. As a result, the U is recognized as a T (thymidine) and C:G is converted to a T:A (adenine) base pair. AID is responsible not only for causing mutations that produce antibody diversity during GC development of B lymphocytes, but also for those that lead to B cell lymphoma.[55] AID must be tightly controlled in B cells to minimize off-target mutations leading to chromosomal translocations and the development of B cell malignancies.[56]

Consistent with the model proposed here, RA influences both AID and the *c-myc* translocation. For instance, RA participates in the regulated expression of several genes essential for B cell activation and differentiation, including AID,[57] and has been found to enhance the expression of AID in immunodeficiency-derived human B cells.[58] *C-myc* also interacts with the retinoic acid receptor-α (RARα) and is recruited to RAR DNA binding sequences (or receptor elements, RAREs) in leukemia cells. This *c-myc*/RARα complex can either activate or repress RARα-dependent targets through a phosphorylation switch. Unphosphorylated *c-myc*/RARα represses the expression of RAR targets required for differentiation, thereby increasing the risk of leukemia malignancy, whereas if *c-myc* is phosphorylated by the kinase Pak2, the *c-myc*/RARα complex activates transcription of those same genes to stimulate differentiation, thus reducing tumor risk.[59]

HIV, EBV and Retinoic Acid

An important role for HIV infection in EBV and BL is also recognized. HIV infection is estimated to increase the likelihood of developing a lymphoma by 60 to 110-fold; moreover, HIV/AIDS-related lymphomas are predominantly B-cell lymphomas. Burkitt's lymphoma is 1000 times more common in HIV patients than in the general population and accounts for up to 40% of HIV-associated lymphomas.[60] The pathogenesis of HIV and the cause of the decline in CD4 T cells remain obscure. Although some studies suggest that vitamin A supplementation is associated with disease improvement, others with disease worsening,[61] dietary intake of vitamin A (and of niacin and zinc) was reported to be significantly associated with progression from HIV to acquired immunodeficiency syndrome (AIDS).[62] The HIV genome also has a retinoic acid receptor element, suggesting that vitamin A may increase HIV replication via interacting with this element. Vitamin A supplementation also increases the differentiation of myeloid and lymphoid cells, which are associated with increased expression of CCR5 receptors, and the latter are essential for attachment of HIV to T-lymphocytes and thus a key co-factor for HIV replication.[63] Dendritic cells (DCs) are important players in HIV infection and dissemination. DCs in the gut produce RA from retinol by oxidation or may take it up from epithelial cell. RA has been shown to increase the DC's ability to enhance HIV infection and may contribute to the rapid spread of HIV in the gut, a major site of HIV replication after mucosal exposure.[64] Thus, HIV infection, like malaria, could be another pathway to EBV infection and BL involving alterations in retinoid metabolism.

Further Reflections

The retinoid toxicity model proposed here suggests that *P. falciparum*, the *Plasmodium* species that causes the most severe form of malaria, is specifically linked to BL because of the ability of the parasite to absorb and utilize higher concentrations of retinoic acid from the host than other species; it also suggests that children are at greater risk of BL because of their increased sensitivity to vitamin A, with daily intakes of 1500 IU/kg body weight reportedly leading to toxicity.[28] It is recalled that hemozoin was not as effective as complete extracts from *P. falciparum* in inducing AID in tonsil B cells from individuals with malaria, suggesting a role for other components.[20] This observation is tentatively explained on the basis that complete extracts from *P. falciparum* would be likely to contain high concentrations of the putative toxin, retinoic acid. The predilection of BL for the jaw and other facial bones of young children may be similarly related to the known adverse effects of hypervitaminosis A on bone.[65]

Testing the Hypothesis

It has been suggested that alterations in retinoid metabolism involving increased RAR expression are importantly involved in the mechanisms underlying the close association between malaria, EBV infection and Burkitt's lymphoma. The model could be tested by studies of retinoid profiles (retinol, retinyl esters and retinoic acid) and RAR expression in plasma and lymphatic tissues of patients with BL and controls. Current treatments for BL have achieved high survival rates, but treatment-related toxicity and immunodeficiency remain major barriers to improving survival among children with BL.[66] Subject to obtaining results consistent with the proposed model, studies could be initiated to determine the efficacy and safety of interventions that affect retinoid metabolism and lower the availability and expression of retinoic acid as potential treatments for BL.

Financial Disclosure or Conflict of Interest

None.

Acknowledgments

We thank Olugbemiga Ekundayo, Ann Moormann and Catherine Ross for their valuable comments on earlier drafts of the paper.

References

1. Burkitt DP. A sarcoma involving the jaws in African children. Br J Surg 1958; 46(197):218–23. 34.
2. Molyneux EM, Rochford R, Griffin B, Newton R, Jackson G, Menon G, Harrison CJ, Israels T, Bailey S. Burkitt's lymphoma. Lancet 2012; 379(9822):1234-44. doi: 10.1016/S0140-6736(11)61177-X.
3. Brady G, MacArthur GJ, Farrell PJ. Epstein-Barr virus and Burkitt lymphoma. Postgrad Med J 2008; 84(993):372–377.
4. God JM, Haque A. Burkitt lymphoma: pathogenesis and immune evasion. J Oncol 2010; 2010:516047. October 5. Doi: 10.1155/2010/16047.
5. Allday MJ. How does Epstein-Barr virus (EBV) complement the activation of Myc in the pathogenesis of Burkitt's lymphoma? Sem Cancer Biol 2009; 19(6):366-376.
6. Kafuko GW, Burkitt DP. Burkitt's lymphoma and malaria. Int J Cancer 1970; 6:1-9.
7. Chêne A, Donati D, Guerreiro-Cacais AO, Levitsky V, Chen Q, Falk KI, Orem J, Kironde F, Wahlgren M, Bejarano MT. A molecular link between malaria and Epstein-Barr virus reactivation. PLOS Pathogens 2007; 3(6):e80. DOI:10.1371/journal.ppat.0030080.
8. Epstein MA, Achong BG, Barr YM, Zajac B, Henle G, Henle W. Morphological and virological investigations on cultured Burkitt tumor lymphoblasts (strain Raji). J Natl Cancer Inst 1966; 37(4):547-59.
9. Magrath I. The pathogenesis of Burkitt's lymphoma. Adv Cancer Res 1990; 55:133-270.
10. Bornkamm GW. Epstein-Barr virus and the pathogenesis of Burkitt's lymphoma: more questions than answers. Int J Cancer 2009; 124(8):1745-1755.
11. Pietersma F, Piriou E, van Baarle D. Immune surveillance of EBV-infected B cells and the development of non-Hodgkin lymphomas in immunocompromised patients. Leukemia and Lymphoma 2008; 49(6):1028-1041.
12. Magrath I. Epidemiology: clues to the pathogenesis of Burkitt lymphoma. Br J Haematol 2012; 156(6):744-56. doi: 10.1111/j.1365-2141.2011.09013.x.

13. Blum KA, Lozanski G, Byrd JC. Adult Burkitt leukemia and lymphoma. Blood 2004; 104:3009–20.
14. Johnston WT, Mutalima N, Sun D, Emmanuel B, Bhatia K, Aka P, Wu X, Borgstein E, Liomba GN, Kamiza S, Mkandawire N, Batumba M, Carpenter LM, Jaffe H, Molyneux EM, Goedert JJ, Soppet D, Newton R, Mbulaiteye SM. Relationship between Plasmodium falciparum malaria prevalence, genetic diversity and endemic Burkitt lymphoma in Malawi. Sci Rep 2014; 4:3741. doi: 10.1038/srep03741.
15. Moormann AM, Snider CJ, Chelimo K. The company malaria keeps: how co-infection with Epstein-Barr virus leads to endemic Burkitt lymphoma. Curr Opin Infect Dis 2011; 24:435-441.
16. Moormann AM, Heller KN, Chelimo K, Embury P, Ploutz-Snyder R, Otieno JA, Oduor M, Münz C, Rochford R. Children with endemic Burkitt lymphoma are deficient in EBNA1-specific IFN-γ T cell responses. Int J Cancer 2009; 124(7):1721-1726.
17. Thorley-Lawson D, Deitsch KW, Duca KA, Torgbor C. The link between Plasmodium falciparum malaria and endemic Burkitt's lymphoma – New insight into a 50-year-old enigma. PLoS Pathog 2016; 12: e1005331.
18. Ramiro AR, Jankovic M, Eisenreich T, Difilippantonio S, Chen-Kiang S, Muramatsu M, Honjo T, Nussenzweig A, Nussenzweig MC. AID is required for c-myc/IgH chromosome translocations in vivo. Cell 2004; 118(4):431-8.
19. Park SR. Activation-induced cytidine deaminase in B cell immunity and cancers. Immune Netw 2012; 12(6):230-9. doi: 10.4110/in.2012.12.6.230. Epub 2012 Dec 31.
20. Torgbor C, Awuah P, Deitsch K, Kalantari P, Duca KA, Thorley-Lawson DA. A multifactorial role for P. falciparum malaria in endemic Burkitt's lymphoma pathogenesis. PLoS Pathog 2014; 10(5): e1004170. doi:10.1371/journal.ppat.1004170
21. Robbiani DF, Deroubaix S, Feldhahn N, Oliveira TY, Callen E, Wang Q, Jankovic M, Silva IT, Rommel PC, Bosque D, Eisenreich T, Nussenzweig A, Nussenzweig MC. Plasmodium infection promotes genomic instability and AID-dependent B Cell lymphoma. Cell 2015; 162(4):727-37. doi: 10.1016/j.cell.2015.07.019.
22. Mizuno Y, Kawazu SI, Kano S, Watanabe N, Matsuura T, Ohtomo H. In-vitro uptake of vitamin A by Plasmodium falciparum. Ann Trop Med Parasitol 2003; 97(3):237-43.
23. Gouado I, Lehman LG, Some IT, Mbouyap Y, Pankoui MJB, Ejoh AR, Tchouanguep MF. Influence of malaria on the serum levels of vitamin

A, zinc and calcium of children in Douala-Cameroon. African Journal of Biotechnology 2007; 6(7): 871-876.
24. Doldo E, Costanza G, Agostinelli S, Tarquini C, Ferlosio A, Arcuri G, Passeri D, Scioli MG, Orlandi A. Vitamin A, cancer treatment and prevention: the new role of cellular retinol binding proteins. Biomed Res Int 2015; 2015:624627. doi: 10.1155/2015/624627.
25. de Oliveira MR. Vitamin A and retinoids as mitochondrial toxicants. Oxid Med Cell Longev 2015; 2015:140267. doi: 10.1155/2015/140267.
26. Theodosiou M, Laudet V, Schubert M. From carrot to clinic: an overview of the retinoic acid signalling pathway. Coll Mol Life Sci 2010; 67:1423-1445.
27. Penniston KL, Tanumihardjo SA. The acute and chronic toxic effects of vitamin A. Am J Clin Nutr 2006; 83:191-201.
28. Schnorr CE, da Silva Morrone M, Simões-Pires A, da Rocha RF, Behr GA, Moreira JC. Vitamin A supplementation in rats under pregnancy and nursing induces behavioral changes and oxidative stress upon striatum and hippocampus of dams and their offspring. Brain Res 2011; 1369:60-73.
29. Leo MA, Lieber CS. New pathway of retinol metabolism in liver microsomes. J Biol Chem 1985; 260:5228-31.
30. Dingle T, Lucy JA. Studies on the mode of action of excess vitamin A. The effect of vitamin A on the stability of the erythrocyte membrane. J. Biochem 1962; 84, 611-621.
31. Mawson AR. The pathogenesis of malaria: A new perspective. Path Global Health 2013; 107(3):122-129.
32 Perrotta S, Nobili B, Rossi F, Criscuolo M, Iolascon A, Di Pinto D, Passaro I, Cennamo L, Oliva A, Ragione DF. Infant hypervitaminosis A causes severe anemia and thrombocytopenia: evidence of a retinol-dependent bone marrow cell growth inhibition. Blood 2002; 99(6):2017-2022.
33. Neves M, Marinho-Dias J, Ribeiro J, Sousa H. Epstein-Barr virus strains and variations: Geographic or disease-specific variants? J Med Virol 2017; 89(3):373-387. doi: 10.1002/jmv.24633.
34. Wolbach SB, Howe PR. Tissue changes following deprivation of fat-soluble A vitamin. J Exp Med 1925; 42:753-77.
35. Wang ZY, Chen Z. Acute promyelocytic leukemia: from highly fatal to highly curable. Blood 2008; 111:2505-2515.
36. Frankel SR, Eardley A, Heller G, Berman E, Miller WH Jr, Dmitrovsky E, Warrell RP Jr. All-trans retinoic acid for acute promyelocytic leukemia. Ann Intern Med 1994; 120:278-286.

37. Su YC, Dunn P, Shih LY, Kuo MC, Chang H, Wu JH, Lin TL, Wang PN, Tang TC, Hung YS. Retinoic acid syndrome in patients following the treatment of acute promyelocytic leukemia with all-trans retinoic acid. Chang Gung Med J 2009; 32:535-42.
38. Bushue N, Wan YJY. Retinoid pathway and cancer therapeutics. Adv Drug Deliv Rev 2010; doi:10.1016/j.addr2010.07.003.
39. Omenn GS, Goodman GE, Thornquist MD, Balmes J, Cullen MR, Glass A, Keogh JP, Meyskens FL, Valanis B, Williams JH, Barnhart S, Hammar S. NEJM 1996; 334: 1150-1155
40. Hennekens CH, Buring JE, Manson JE, Stampfer M, Rosner B, Cook NR, Belanger C, LaMotte F, Gaziano JM, Ridker PM, Willett W, Peto R. Lack of effect of long-term supplementation with beta carotene on the incidence of malignant neoplasms and cardiovascular disease. NEJM 1996; 334, 1145-1149.
41. Fritz H, Kennedy D, Fergusson D, Fernandes R, Doucette S, Cooley K, Seely A, Sagar S, Wong R, Seely D. Vitamin A and retinoid derivatives for lung cancer: a systematic review and meta-analysis. PLoS ONE 2011; 6(6): e21107. doi:10.1371/journal.pone.0021107
42. Albahrani AA, Greaves RF. Fat-soluble vitamins: clinical indications and current challenges for chromatographic measurement. Clin Biochem Rev 2016; 37(1):27-47.
43. Pasquali MA, Schnorr CE, Feistauer LB, Gelain DP, Moreira JC. Vitamin A supplementation to pregnant and breastfeeding female rats induces oxidative stress in the neonatal lung. Reprod Toxicol 2010; 30(3):452-6.
44. Zanotto-Filho A, Schröder F, Moreira JCF. Differential effects of retinol and retinoic acid on cell proliferation: a role for reactive species and redox-dependent mechanisms in retinol supplementation. Free Radical Res 2008; 42:778-788.
45. Møllersen L, Paulsen JE, Olstørn HB, Knutsen HK, Alexander J. Dietary retinoic acid supplementation stimulates intestinal tumour formation and growth in multiple intestinal neoplasia (Min)/+ mice. Carcinogenesis 2004; 25:149-53.
46. Tammariello AE, Milner JA. Mouse models for unraveling the importance of diet in colon cancer prevention. J Nutr Biochem 2010; 21(2):77-88. doi: 10.1016/j.jnutbio.2009.09.014.
47. Bjelakovic G, Nikolova D, Gluud LL, Simonetti RG, Gluud C. Mortality in randomized trials of antioxidant supplements for primary and secondary prevention: systematic review and meta-analysis. JAMA 2007; 297:842-57.

48. Ghazal P, LeBlanc JF, Angulo A. Vitamin A regulation of viral growth. Rev Med Virol 1997; 7:21-34.
49. Angulo A, Suto C, Boehm MF, Heyman RA, Ghazal P. Retinoid activation of retinoic acid receptors but not of retinoid X receptors promotes cellular differentiation and replication of human cytomegalovirus in embryonal cells. J Virol 1995; 69:3831–3837.
50. Jones RJ, Dickerson S, Bhende PM, Delecluse HJ, Kenney SC. Epstein-Barr virus lytic infection induces retinoic acid-responsive genes through induction of a retinol-metabolizing enzyme, DHRS9. J BiolChem 2007;282(11):8317-24.
51. Yunusa UM, Attah C Vitamin A and Immunity: A Review Chemistry Research Journal, 2016, 1(1):44-49. http://chemrj.org/download/vol-1-iss-1-2016/chemrj0101006.pdf
52. Ross AC, Chen Q, Ma Y. Vitamin A and retinoic acid in the regulation of B-cell development and antibody production. Vitam Horm 2011; 86:103-26.
53. Mbulaiteye SM. Burkett's lymphoma: beyond discoveries. Infect Agent Cancer 2013; 8(1):35. Doi: 10.1186/1750-9378-8-35.
54. Hoffman R. Hematology: basic principles and practice (PDF) (5th ed.). Philadelphia, PA: Churchill Livingstone/Elsevier. 2009: 1304–1305. ISBN 978-0-443-06715-0.
55. Lenz G, Staudt LM. Aggressive lymphomas. N Engl J Med 2010; 362(15): 1417–29. doi:10.1056/NEJMra0807082. PMID 20393178.
56. Casellas R, Basu U, Yewdell WT, Chaudhuri J, Robbiani DF, Di Noia JM. Mutations, kataegis and translocations in B cells: understanding AID promiscuous activity. Nat Rev Immunol 2016; 16(3):164-76. doi: 10.1038/nri.2016.2. Epub 2016 Feb 22.
57. Chen Q, Mosovsky KL, Ross AC. Retinoic acid and α-galactosylceramide regulate the expression of costimulatory receptors and transcription factors responsible for B cell activation and differentiation. Immunobiology 2013; 218(12):1477-87. doi: 10.1016/j.imbio.2013.05.003. Epub 2013 May 20.
58. Indrevær RL, Moskaug JØ, Paur I, Bøhn SK, Jørgensen SF, Blomhoff R, Aukrust P, Fevang B, Blomhoff HK. IRF4 Is a critical gene in retinoic acid-mediated plasma cell formation and is deregulated in common variable immunodeficiency-derived B Cells. J Immunol 2015; 195(6):2601-11. doi: 10.4049/jimmunol.1500250.
59. Uribesalgo I, Benitah SA, Di Croce L. From oncogene to tumor suppressor: The dual role of Myc in leukemia. Cell Cycle 2012; 11(9):1757-64.

60. Mahe E, Ross C, Sur M. Lymphoproliferative lesions in the setting of HIV infection: a five-year retrospective case series and review. Patholog Res Int 2011; 2011:618760; doi:10:4061/2011/618760
61. Chandrasekhar A, Gupta A. Nutrition and disease progression pre–highly active antiretroviral therapy (HAART) and post-HAART: can good nutrition delay time to HAART and affect response to HAART? Am J Clin Nutr 2011;
94(6):1703S-1715S. doi:10.3945/ajcn.111.019018.
62. Tang AM, Graham NM, Kirby AJ, McCall LD, Willett WC, Saah AJ. Dietary micronutrient intake and risk of progression to acquired immunodeficiency syndrome (AIDS) in human immunodeficiency virus type 1 (HIV-1)-infected homosexual men. Am J Epidemiol 1993; 138(11):937-51.
63. Mehta S, Fawzi W. Effects of vitamins, including vitamin A, on HIV/AIDS patients. Vitam Horm 2007; 75:355-83.
64. Guerra-Pérez N, Frank I, Veglia F, Aravantinou M, Goode D, Blanchard JL, Gettie A, Robbiani M, Martinelli E. Retinoic acid imprints a mucosal-like phenotype on dendritic cells with an increased ability to fuel HIV-1 infection. J Immunol 2015; 194(5):2415-23. doi: 10.4049/jimmunol.1402623.
65. Barker ME, Blumsohn A. Is vitamin A consumption a risk factor for osteoporotic fracture? Proc Nutr Soc 2003; 62 (4): 845–50. doi:10.1079/PNS2003306.
66. Moormann AM, Skiles JL, Otieno JA, Buckle GC, Vik TA. Optimal management of endemic Burkitt lymphoma: a holistic approach mindful of limited resources. Blood and Lymphatic Cancer: Targets and Therapy 2014:4 91–99.

4

DETERMINING THE IMPACT OF A WEST CENTRAL AFRICAN-STYLE DIET ON AFRICAN AMERICANS WITH TYPE 2 DIABETES AND HYPERTENSION: A QUASI-EXPERIMENTAL STUDY

(RFA-RM-21-022 – The NIH Common Fund's New Funding Opportunity: TRANSFORMATIVE RESEARCH TO ADDRESS HEALTH DISPARITIES)
May 11, 2021

Abstract

Background – African Americans are at increased risk of type 2 diabetes mellitus (T2DM) and hypertension, which affect over a third of U.S. adults. These closely overlapping conditions track each other from an early age and over time. Growing evidence suggests a common etiopathogenesis in nonalcoholic fatty liver disease (NAFLD). Insulin acts on the liver both to take up glucose and to mobilize and secrete vitamin A. NAFLD impairs insulin-induced glucose uptake, leading to insulin resistance and to the spillage of stored vitamin A compounds (retinoids) into the circulation in toxic concentrations. This is followed over time by kidney damage, worsening hypertension, and the secondary consequences of diabetes. The theory is proposed that the susceptibility of people of West Central African descent to these conditions is related to evolutionary physiological adaptations to the original environment of potentially lethal endemic parasitism, one of which is a tendency towards reduced enzymatic catabolism of vitamin A. As a result, retinoids accumulate to sub-toxic levels and weaken the parasite, thereby protecting against severe malaria. This represented a successful adaptation to the environment. However, in North America, where the diet is mainly dairy-based and lethal parasites are absent, African Americans are especially susceptible to conditions associated with retinoid toxicity, which include T2DM and hypertension. Traditional West Central African diets are low in preformed vitamin A and high in vitamin A-absorbing fiber. Adoption of such diets could therefore help to prevent and treat these diseases. Specific Aims: To test the key hypothesis: that adoption of a traditional West Central African-style diet significantly reduces HgA1c and blood pressure, due to a decreased percentage of retinyl esters to total vitamin A, after adjusting for potential confounding factors. Methods: A before-and-after quasi-experimental study design, with participants serving as their own controls. Subject to IRB approval, three groups of 20 consenting adults diagnosed with T2DM and hypertension, successively trained in the cuisine, will adopt it for 12 weeks. Access to food items on the diet will be provided locally by … Farms. Expected Results and Significance: Adherence to the diet is expected to lead to clinically significant reductions in HbA1c and blood pressure via the normalization of retinoid concentration profiles. Long-term adherence to the diet could lower the risk of progression to cardiovascular diseases and stroke and have a transformative impact as a population-based strategy for reducing and even eliminating disparities in other chronic diseases.

Specific Aims

Significance, Innovation, and Impact

The proposed study is designed to determine the impact of a West Central African-style diet on African American adults diagnosed with type 2 diabetes mellitus (T2DM) and hypertension. The study is based on a new theory of the pathogenesis and the susceptibility of people of West Central African descent to these diseases. T2DM and hypertension closely overlap and track each other over time and from an early age, including preterm birth, suggesting a common etiology. While T2DM is attributed primarily to insulin resistance and disturbed glucose homeostasis, growing evidence suggests that a common initiating cause of T2DM and hypertension is nonalcoholic fatty liver disease (NAFLD). Insulin acts on the liver both to take up glucose from the circulation and to mobilize and secrete vitamin A. It is hypothesized that NAFLD impairs the actions of insulin, resulting in insulin resistance and in the spillage of stored retinoid compounds into the circulation in toxic concentrations. Over time, this leads to kidney and pancreatic damage, worsening hypertension, and the secondary consequences of diabetes via retinoid toxicity-induced endothelial and mitochondrial dysfunction and apoptosis. African Americans may prone to these conditions due to higher levels of retinoids in certain tissues and to a tendency toward reduced cytochrome (CYP26) enzymatic catabolism of retinoic acid, causing it to accumulate to sub-toxic levels. In the original environment this served the useful purpose of weakening the parasite, thereby reducing the risk of severe malaria. Based on these concepts, adoption of a West Central African-style diet, which is low in preformed vitamin A and high in vitamin A-absorbing fiber, could reverse T2DM and hypertension and lower the risk of progression to chronic diseases and stroke. The expected successful outcome of this project will be improved glucose metabolism and blood pressure. Long-term, adoption of the diet could have a transformational impact on understanding the pathogenesis and management of these conditions, leading to the reduction and even elimination of disparities in T2DM and hypertension and to the prevention of related diseases in the broader community.

Insight and Rationale

Disparities in healthcare affecting African Americans remain rooted in structural racism and discrimination and the legacy of the Jim Crow era. A contributory role for additional factors in overall health is suggested by the observation that increased susceptibility to certain diseases is paralleled by reduced risks of other diseases; notably malaria, dengue, yellow fever, and NAFLD. It is proposed that this profile has arisen from evolutionary physiological adaptations to the sub-Saharan African environment. Like the hemoglobinopathies sickle cell trait and G6PD deficiency, they are related to exposure to potentially lethal endemic parasitism. It is suggested that the initiating stimulus for these adaptations is the selective absorption of vitamin A from the human host by *Plasmodia* and its subsequent use in parasite reproduction and disease pathogenesis. Over the course of millennia these adaptations led to 1) the sequestering vitamin A away from the liver to other organs, to reduce its accessibility to the parasite; and 2) to reduced vitamin A catabolism, causing it to accumulate to toxic concentrations and weaken the parasite. These adaptations were successful in reducing the risk of severe malaria. However, in North America, where lethal parasites are absent and the diet is high in vitamin A, retinoids may accumulate in specific tissues such as the kidney, pancreas, and heart, contributing to disease risks and health disparities affecting African Americans. Retinoid toxicity is increasingly linked to numerous acute and chronic conditions via mitochondrial dysfunction and apoptosis. While much research is needed to test and explore its implications, the theory suggests that adoption of traditional West Central African-style diets may hold promise not only for disease management and treatment but as a transformative concept and strategy that could lead to improved overall health and longevity and to major reductions in health disparities.

Research Strategy

Overview of Research Project

The research team and partners propose to test the hypothesis that adoption of a West Central African-style diet for 12 weeks will have a significant positive impact on the overall health of African American adults diagnosed with T2DM and hypertension, leading to clinically significant reductions in HgA1c and blood pressure due to significant changes in retinoid concentration profiles (i.e., lowered retinoic acid concentrations and percent retinyl esters to total vitamin A), after controlling for potential confounding factors. This before-and-after quasi-experimental study will involve three groups of 20 patient volunteers who will be successively trained in the cuisine of West Central Africa, provided with access to the appropriate foodstuffs, and will adhere to the diet for 12 weeks.

State-of-the-art in the Field of Health Disparities and Metabolic Disorders and How the Proposed Study and Program will Transform the Field. The fundamental new insight driving this project.

Disparities in healthcare affecting African Americans remain rooted in the pervasive impact of structural racism and discrimination, resulting in limited quality and access to healthcare, education, and housing, as well as lower incomes and stress related to experiences of racial prejudice (Institute of Medicine, 2002; Williams et al., 2019). The legacy of 400 years of slavery, violent repression and stress suffered by African Americans in the struggle for equality cannot be underestimated, and it continues to affect individuals, families, and the entire community (Braveman and Gottlieb, 2014; deShazo, 2018). Certain observations on the overall health of people of West Central African descent suggest a contributory role for additional factors. For instance, compared to white physicians, black physicians have a higher rate and an earlier onset of heart disease, higher disease fatality rates (52% vs. 9%), and twofold higher rates of diabetes and hypertension (Thomas et al., 1997). African American youths with type 1 diabetes also have higher glycated hemoglobin (HbA1c) levels after adjustment for many factors, and higher rates of severe hypoglycemia and ketoacidosis. They also require higher doses of insulin per body weight and have a higher rate of hypertension (Redondo et al., 2018). Although more susceptible to certain diseases and conditions than people of European descent, people of West Central African descent are less susceptible to other diseases, including severe malaria, dengue, yellow fever, and nonalcoholic fatty liver disease. These observations suggest a potential role for nutrition and genetic factors.

The Potentially Dramatic Beneficial Impact of a Traditional West Central African Diet on African American Adults

In a study in which 20 rural South Africans and 20 African Americans switched diets for two weeks, the Africans consumed American food, consisting mainly of meat and cheese, while the African Americans consumed the African diet, which is high in fiber and low in fat and consists of vegetables, beans, cornmeal, and little meat. Africans on the American diet quickly developed intestinal mucosal inflammation and a cytokine profile in the gut related to intestinal cancer. In contrast, when African Americans were placed on a traditional African diet their existing intestinal inflammation disappeared and produced butyrate, a fatty acid known to protect against colon cancer (O'Keefe et al, 1997). These effects suggest a potential toxin in the U.S. diet to which people of West Central African descent are especially sensitive. It is proposed that this toxin is vitamin A.

The Fundamental New Insight Driving this Project

No single diet is healthy for all human beings, and both diets and physiologies have evolved together over millennia as successful adaptations to environmental challenges and resources. For instance, dairy-based diets and physiological adaptations to cow milk proteins have evolved in the case of northern Europeans, exposed to and dependent upon grazing animals. In the case of people of West Central African descent, mainly plant-based diets have evolved partly as adaptations to potentially lethal endemic parasitism, along with physiological adaptations that included hemoglobinopathies but went beyond them to include susceptibilities to other chronic diseases (Mawson, 2021). These were adaptations to the selective absorption of vitamin A from the human host (Mizuno et al., 2003) and to its use in parasite reproduction and disease pathogenesis. Vitamin A in higher concentration is cytotoxic, prooxidant, mutagenic, and teratogenic and causes mitochondrial dysfunction and apoptosis (Oliveiro et al., 2015). Upon their emergence from the liver, the merozoite-stage malaria parasite is hypothesized to use its absorbed vitamin A as a membrane destabilizer to enter and reproduce in the red blood cells. At their demise, the damaged cells release the vitamin A into the circulation, causing the signs and symptoms of the disease as endogenous manifestations of hypervitaminosis A (Mawson, 2013). This hypothesis is supported by a recent study showing, as predicted, that patients with Plasmodium vivax malaria have low concentrations of retinol but high concentrations of retinoic acid, the major and potentially more toxic metabolite of retinol (Na et al., 2019).

The evolutionary adaptations in question included 1) sequestering of vitamin A away from the liver, where it is mainly stored, to other organs, to reduce its access to the parasite; and 2) reducing the CYP26 enzymatic catabolism of vitamin A, causing it to accumulate and weaken the parasite, thereby lowering the risk of severe disease. These adaptations were successful in the original environment, enhancing health and longevity, but in North America, where lethal parasitism is absent and diets are mainly dairy-based, people of West Central African descent are at increased risk of vitamin A toxicity-related diseases; these include cardiovascular and metabolic diseases, cancer, and teratogenesis, and increasingly implicate T2DM. The hypothesized sequestering of vitamin A away from the liver to other organs, including the kidney, pancreas, and heart, could trigger inflammation and contribute to increased risks of metabolic disorders, vascular disease, and other organ-specific diseases. The hypothesized adaptation of reduced CYP26 catabolism of retinoic acid could also contribute to increased risks of liver damage and the subsequent spillage and redistribution of stored retinoids to other organs in toxic concentrations. African Americans, it is suggested, are especially sensitive to the toxic effects of vitamin A but not to saturated fat, the latter of which has obscured the role of vitamin A and has been mistakenly linked to heart disease and caused an upheaval in global nutrition for over 60 years, leading to the worldwide epidemics of obesity, fatty liver disease, and diabetes (Begley, 2017). The theory is depicted in the diagram below.

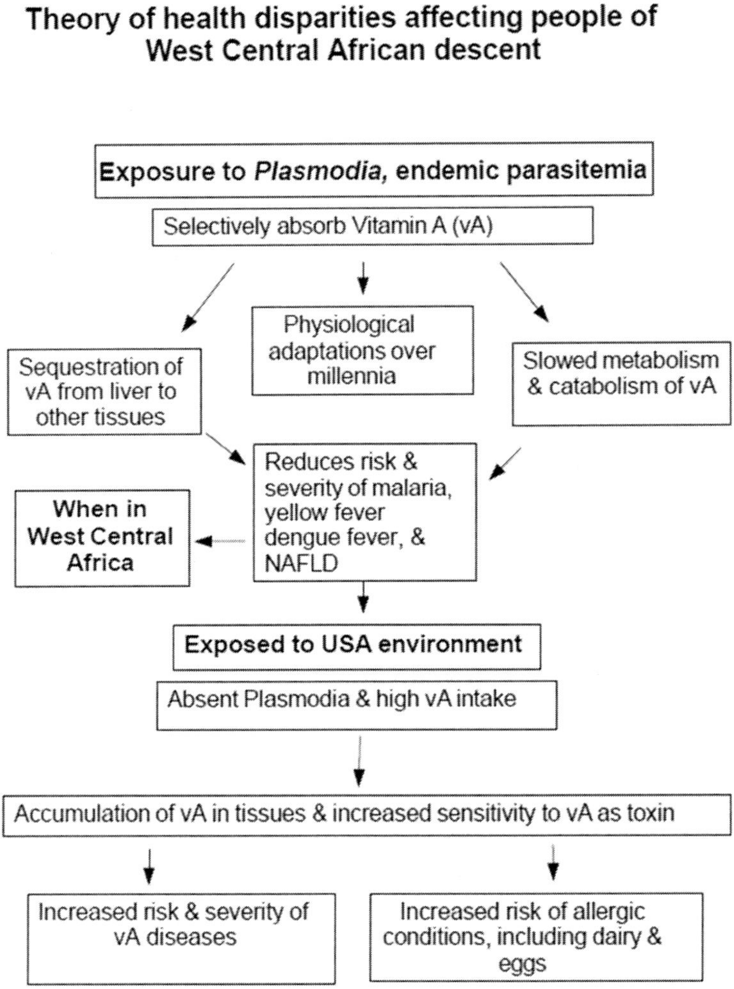

Figure. Vitamin A toxicity hypothesis of health disparities affecting people of West Central African descent in the US.

Malaria parasites selectively absorb vitamin A and spend over a week in the liver, the main storage site of vitamin A. Endemic exposure to Plasmodia and other common parasites in the original environment is hypothesized to have led to evolutionary adaptations involving 1) the sequestration of vitamin A from the liver to subcutaneous adipose and other tissues, to reduce its accessibility to the parasite; and 2) reduced vitamin A enzymatic metabolism and catabolism, causing it to accumulate to sub-toxic concentrations and weaken the parasite, thereby reducing the risk of severe disease. These adaptations may have reduced the severity of malaria, yellow fever, dengue, and the risk of NAFLD in people of West Central African descent. However, in North America, where major parasites are absent and high vitamin A-containing diets are the norm, these adaptations may cause vitamin A to accumulate in the tissues, thereby increasing the risk and severity of many chronic diseases. They may also have led to an enhanced sensitivity to vitamin A as a cellular toxin, and increased risks of allergy. These adaptations may be contributing to the emergence of a similar health profile in West Central Africans as western diets are increasingly adopted.

These considerations suggest that adoption of traditional West Central African-style diets that are low in preformed vitamin A and high in vitamin A-absorbing fiber may prove to be an effective adjunct method for treating T2DM and hypertension (and other diseases that are increasingly linked to vitamin A toxicity) and as a population-based strategy for overall health maintenance and longevity. Although these diets are mainly plant-based, they tend to be heavily spiced and are often rich in saturated fat (Congolese food and cultural profile: dietetic consultation guide. State of Queensland, 2015. https://metrosouth.health.qld.gov.au/sites/default/files/profile_congolese_dietetic.pdf). It should be noted that the suggested role of vitamin A toxicity in T2DM is relatively novel and controversial (e.g., Trasino and Gudas, 2015). Our study will shed light on this critical question. Vitamin A is usually assessed in terms of serum retinol, which is tightly controlled and varies little over a wide range of dietary intake; it can even be low in the blood in the presence of vitamin A toxicity related to dietary or supplement intake, due to impaired mobilization and secretion from the liver. The accepted indicator of vitamin A toxicity in adults – percent retinyl esters >10% as a fraction of total vitamin A (retinyl esters plus retinol) (Tanumihardjo et al., 2016) has very seldom been measured in clinical studies. Thanks to [a member of the research team] we will be able to assess this indicator in our study in patients with T2DM and hypertension before, during and after the diet.

Innovation – The proposed study is novel in conception compared to current approaches, paradigms, practices, and theoretical perspectives. No such study has been conducted to date, to our knowledge. It is also transformational in its implications for health and for reducing disparities in health. The theory explains the susceptibility of African Americans to T2DM and hypertension as related to the same mechanisms that underlie the causes of the diseases themselves; and that T2DM and hypertension stem from a common origin in disturbed liver function and vitamin A metabolism and resulting vitamin A toxicity.

Banting and Best's discovery of insulin in 1921-1922 and their demonstration of its therapeutic effect in dogs and humans was a momentous advance in the history of medicine. Yet it was soon apparent that that the etiology was more complex than mere destruction of islet tissue; and understanding the action of insulin was an exceedingly complex problem involving the elucidation of the intermediary metabolism not only of carbohydrate but of protein and fat (Travis and Sayers, 1970). Today, 100 years after Banting and Best's discovery, the etiology of diabetes mellitus is still uncertain, and prevention remains a distant prospect. Since the introduction of insulin therapy in 1921 the death rate from diabetic ketoacidosis has dramatically fallen. However, there are numerous unexplained and debilitating long-term complications of the disease, including neuropathy, nephropathy, retinopathy, cataract, and atherosclerosis.

The continuing focus of most research is on attempts to understand and correct the disturbances in glucose metabolism that result from the disease and that are assumed to have a primary role in the long-term complications of diabetes (Aoki et al., 1993). Relatively little attention is given to the question of the initiating cause of the beta-cell damage and whether this same initiating factor (or factors), as opposed to the more obvious hyperglycemia, may be responsible for the later complications of the disease. The suggestion here is that the etiopathogenesis and long-term complications of diabetes mellitus include the toxic effects of prolonged exposure to excessive concentrations of vitamin A and its metabolites, and a central role is played by impaired liver function, in which the initial lesion to the beta-cells may be due to excess exposure to circulating retinoids (in particular, retinyl esters and retinoic acid).

Although African Americans are less prone to fatty liver disease than European Americans, they are more prone to develop advanced liver disease (Liu et al., 2011). This paradoxical observation, that AAs are prone to advanced liver disease despite lower levels of liver fat, may be due to the postulated tendency toward reduced vA metabolism and hence increased vA accumulation and potential toxicity. Even with lower levels of liver fat, African Americans may be more sensitive to vitamin A as a toxin and more likely to experience inflammatory changes, e.g., in the liver, indicated by increased liver enzymes, as well as more prone to obesity, hypertension, and diabetes and to severe manifestations of these conditions. In summary, it is suggested that people of West Central African descent are prone to certain chronic diseases, and more severe disease, including fatty liver and diabetes, from which they were originally protected, due to vitamin A-rich North American diets and increased sensitivity to vA as a toxin, resulting from its lower metabolism, catabolism, and greater accumulation.

Approach

This research grant application provides the underlying logic and rationale for pursuing the proposed scientific aims and addresses potential challenges and limitations.

Key Research Questions

The objectives of the dietary intervention study are: 1) To determine the effectiveness of a traditional West Central African-style diet in reducing hemoglobin A1c (HgA1c) in African American adults diagnosed with T2DM and hypertension. 2) To determine whether the decline in HbA1c associated with the diet is due to reductions in percent retinyl esters to total vitamin A (retinyl esters plus retinol) and the concentration of retinoic acid, after controlling for C-reactive protein, anthropometric measures, and changes in medication.

Study Design

A before-and-after quasi-experimental study design is proposed, with a total of 60 participants serving as their own controls. The literature on interventional studies shows that randomized controlled trials (RCTs) are not always suitable in studies of diet and chronic disease, as dietary intake is complex and difficult to study with the use of a linear drug trial approach (Satija et al., 2015). Issues such as compliance and blinding render a RCT design difficult and infeasible in the present context. Our decision to adopt a quasi-experimental design will allow every participant to experience the diet and be tested before, during, and after 12 weeks on the diet. As a result, problems will be eliminated arising from interaction between the experimental and control groups and from perceived participant unfairness in assignments and possible attempts on the part of controls to duplicate exposure to the intervention, which could undermine the integrity of the study.

Participants

Three groups of 20 volunteers, totaling 60 African Americans ages 18 and older, with equal numbers of males and females, diagnosed with T2DM and hypertension will be recruited.

Dietary Intervention Training

Instruction in the diet will be provided by an experienced chef, Nigerian by birth and the owner of several restaurants. The training will allow participants to discover the major foods involved in West Central African cuisine and demonstrate how to prepare meals with them. The diet includes leafy greens, tubers such as yams, nuts, rice, colorful fruits and vegetables, healthy oils, whole grains, fish, eggs, poultry, yogurt, marinades, and sauces made with herbs and spices. The foods are low in processed sugar but include meat and sweets. Muscle meat itself is low in preformed vitamin A. Participants will be encouraged to share what they have learned with family members and friends by jointly preparing West Central African-style meals after each session.

Access to Foodstuffs for the Training and the Diet

Participants will be provided with vouchers to obtain the needed items from [a local farm].

Selected References

Aoki TT, Benbarka MM, Okimura MC, Arcangeli, Walter RM Jr, Wilson LD, Truong MP, Barber AR, Kumagai LF. Long-term intermittent intravenous insulin therapy and type 1 diabetes mellitus. Lancet 1993; 342:515-518.

Begley S. Records found in dusty basement undermine decades of dietary advice: Raw data from a 40-year-old study raises new questions about fats. Sci Am 2017, April 19. https://www.scientificamerican.com/article/records-found-in-dusty-basement-undermine-decades-of-dietary-advice/.

Bhurtyal A. Vitamin A supplementation. From fiasco to scandal. World Nutrition 2016; 7(1-3):117-145.

Blaner WS. Vitamin A signaling and homeostasis in obesity, diabetes, and metabolic disorders. Pharmacol Ther 2019; 197:153-178. https://doi.org/10.1016/j.pharmthera.2019.01.006

Braveman P, Gottlieb L. The social determinants of health: It's time to consider the causes of the causes. Public Health Rep 2014;129(2):19–31.

de Oliveira MR. Vitamin A and retinoids as mitochondrial toxicants. Oxid Med Cell Longev 2015; 2015:140267. doi:10.1155/2015/140267.

deShazo RD (ed). The Racial Divide in American Medicine: Black Physicians and the Struggle for Justice in Health Care. University Press of Mississippi, Jackson, 2018.

Di Masi A, Leboffe L, De Marinis E, Pagano F, Cicconi L, Rochette-Egly C, Lo-Coco F, Ascenzi P, Nervib C. Retinoic acid receptors: From molecular mechanisms to cancer therapy. Molecular Aspects of Medicine 2015; 41:1-115. https://doi.org/10.1016/j.mam.2014.12.003

Harris J. High on the Hog: A Culinary Journey from Africa to America. First edition. Bloomsbury: New York, NY, 2011.

Huk DJ, Harriet L, Hammond HL, Kegechika H, Lincoln J Increased dietary intake of vitamin A promotes aortic valve calcification in vivo. Arterioscler Thromb Vasc Biol 2013; 33(2):285–293; doi: 10.1161/ATVBAHA.112.3003888

Institute of Medicine (IOM). Unequal Treatment: confronting racial and ethnic disparities in health care. Washington, DC: National Academies Press, 2002.

Liu J, Fox CS, Hickson D, Bidulescu A, Carr JJ, Taylor HA. Fatty liver, abdominal visceral fat, and cardiometabolic risk factors: the Jackson Heart Study. Arterioscler Thromb Vasc Biol 2011; 31(11):2715-22. doi: 10.1161/ATVBAHA.111.234062.

Mizuno Y, Kawazu SI, Kano S, Watanabe N, Matsuura T, Ohtomo H. *In-vitro* uptake of vitamin A by *Plasmodium falciparum*. Ann Trop Med Parasitol 2003; 97:237–43. [PubMed] [Google Scholar]

Mawson AR. The pathogenesis of malaria: a new perspective. Pathog Glob Health 2013; 107(3):122-9. doi: 10.1179/2047773213Y.0000000084).

Mawson AR. Understanding the health profile of people of West Central African descent in the United States: A New Perspective. (Submitted to Am J Med Sci, April 2021). [Under consideration by Evolutionary Applications, 2023].

Na J, Khan A, Kim JK, Wadood A, Choe YL, Walker DI, Jones DP, Lim CS, Park YH. Discovery of metabolic alterations in the serum of patients infected with Plasmodium spp. by high-resolution metabolomics. Metabolomics. 2019 Dec 23;16(1):9. doi: 10.1007/s11306-019-1630-2. PMID: 31872321.

O'Keefe SJ, Li JV, Lahti L, Ou J, Carbonero F, Mohammed K, Posma JM, Kinross J, Wahl E, Ruder E, Vipperla K, Naidoo V, Mtshali L, Tims S, Puylaert PG, DeLany J, Krasinskas A, Benefiel AC, Kaseb HO, Newton K, Nicholson JK, de Vos WM, Gaskins HR, Zoetendal EG. Fat, fibre and cancer risk in African Americans and rural Africans. Nat Commun 2015; 6: 6342. doi: 10.1038/ncomms7342.

Redondo MJ, Libman I, Cheng P, Kollman C, Tosur M, Gal RL, Bacha F, Klingensmith GJ, Clements M. Racial/ethnic minority youth with recent-onset Type 1 diabetes have poor prognostic factors. Diabetes Care 2018; 41(5):1017-1024; DOI: 10.2337/dc17-2335

Satija A, Yu E, Willett WC, Hu FB. Understanding nutritional epidemiology and its role in policy. Adv Nutr 2015; 6(1):5-18. Published 2015 Jan 15. doi:10.3945/an.114.007492.

Tanumihardjo SA, Russell RM, Stephensen CB, et al. Biomarkers of Nutrition for Development (BOND)-Vitamin A Review. J Nutr. 2016;146(9):1816S-48S. doi:10.3945/jn.115.229708.

Thomas J, Thomas DJ, Pearson T, Klag M, Mead L. Cardiovascular disease in African American and white physicians: the Meharry Cohort and Meharry-Hopkins Cohort Studies. J Health Care Poor Underserved. 1997 Aug;8(3):270-83; discussion 284. doi: 10.1353/hpu.2010.0526. PMID: 9253218.

Trasino SE, Gudas LJ. Vitamin A: a missing link in diabetes? Diabetes Manag (Lond). 2015; 5(5):359-367. doi: 10.2217/dmt.15.30. PMID: 26535059; PMCID: PMC4623591.

Travis RH, Sayers G. Insulin and oral hypoglycemic drugs. In Goodman LS, Gilman A (eds.), The Pharmacological Basis of Therapeutics, Fourth Edition. New York: Macmillan, 1970, pp. 1581-1603.

Williams DR, Lawrence JA, Davis BA. Racism and health: evidence and needed research. Ann Rev Public Health 2019; 40(1):105-125.

Willett W. Commentary: Dietary diaries versus food frequency questionnaires—a case of undigestible data. Int J Epidemiol 2001; 30(2):317–319, https://doi.org/10.1093/ije/30.2.317

5

AFRICAN AMERICANS ARE AT HIGH RISK OF SEVERE ILLNESS FROM COVID-19 WHEREAS WEST CENTRAL AFRICANS ARE A VERY LOW RISK: EXPLAINING THE CONUNDRUM

Anthony R. Mawson, DrPH, MA
February 27, 2023

Abstract

African Americans are at high risk of severe illness and death from COVID-19. In stark contrast, West Central Africans are at very low risk. The explanation proposed for this conundrum is based on a theory involving three interacting factors in which a central role is played by vitamin A: 1) the nature of the SARS-CoV-2 virus, which has a marked tropism for the biliary tract and liver and has been hypothesized by the author and colleagues to cause the signs and symptoms of COVID-19 via the release of stored retinyl esters into the circulation in toxic concentrations; 2) hypothesized evolutionary physiological adaptations to the ancestral environment of sub-Saharan Africa, which may protect people of West Central African descent from *Plasmodium falciparum* (the latter of which selectively absorbs vitamin A from the liver) and from COVID-19; and 3) the different microbial and dietary environments of West Central Africa and of North America: those of West Central Africa reduce the risk of severe COVID-19 disease whereas those of North America increase it, particularly in African Americans. People of West Central African descent may be more sensitive to vitamin A as a toxin than people of northern European descent, and disparities in the outcomes of COVID-19 and of many chronic inflammatory diseases are conjectured to be due partly to over-expression of the same retinoid-related mechanisms responsible for these diseases in general. The vitamin A toxicity hypothesis suggests that adoption of traditional or modified West Central African-style diets could help in prevention and treatment, since the diets are low in preformed vitamin A and high in vitamin A-absorbing fiber.

High rates of severe COVID-19 in African Americans

African Americans have been adversely affected by the COVID-19 pandemic in terms of age-adjusted rates of severe disease, hospitalization, and death compared to European Americans, particularly during surges of the pandemic. Vaccination rates were lower for African and Hispanic Americans in the initial phases of the vaccine rollout, but they increased over time and were not markedly different from those of European Americans. About 50% of African Americans received at least one dose of a vaccine compared to 56% of European Americans.[1] These findings were confirmed in a separate study of racial disparities in COVID-19 mortality in Michigan, based on individual-linked death certificate and surveillance data. After adjustment for demographic and underlying health characteristics, African Americans were 3·6 times more likely to die than European Americans ($p<0.001$); for those under age 65 without comorbidities the mortality rate of African Americans was 12·6 times higher than that of European Americans ($p<0.001$).[2]

Low rates in West Central Africans

The reverse picture has been observed in West Central African countries: death rates from COVID-19 were markedly lower than those of other countries.[3] With a population of more than one billion people, Africa has been far less adversely affected by the pandemic than the Americas, Europe and Asia in terms of severe morbidity and mortality.[4] Factors believed to have contributed to lower death rates in Africa include the much lower age of the population in most African countries and the fact that most COVID-related deaths occurred in people aged 65 and older. The median age in sub-Saharan Africa is 18 years whereas median ages in North and South America, Europe and Asia range from age 32 to 43.[5] Another factor is lower rates of chronic diseases such as diabetes, chronic respiratory diseases, obesity, and hypertension in sub-Saharan Africa. These diseases increase risks of complications from SARS-CoV-2 infection.[6] Conversely, while low COVID vaccination rates could have increased COVID-19-related infections and deaths, only 24.4% percent of the population in Africa had received at least one dose of a COVID-19 vaccine by July 2022, compared to the global average of 69%.[7]

According to a synthesis of 151 studies on seroprevalence in Africa between January 2020 and December 2021, over two-thirds of Africans had been infected by SARS-CoV-2, and exposure to the virus rose sharply following the emergence of the Beta and Delta variants. Seroprevalence rates varied widely in Africa and appeared to be highest in Eastern, Western and Central African regions.[8] Yet these regions are distinct from other regions of Africa in having high rates of asymptomatic cases, 67% having no symptoms. These low rates of severe illness, hospitalization, and death from COVID-19 in West and Central Africa have remained unexplained. The Beta, Delta and Omicron variants ravaged South Africa, yet much of the rest of the continent did not record similar death tolls. South Africa is the only country in sub-Saharan Africa to record high COVID-19 infection and death rates.[9]

Explaining differences in severe morbidity and death rates from COVID-19 in African Americans compared to West Central Africans

These differences are tentatively explained on the basis of a theory involving three interacting factors in which a central role is played by vitamin A: 1) the nature of the disease, which has a marked tropism for the biliary tract, causing damage to the bile ducts and hepatocytes, potentially leading to liver decompensation and to the myriad signs and symptoms of COVID-19 as an endogenous form of hypervitaminosis A; 2) hypothesized evolutionary physiological adaptations to *Plasmodium falciparum* and other microbial exposures in the ancestral environment, which may serve to protect people of West Central African descent from severe malaria and from severe COVID-19; and 3) the impact of different microbial and dietary environments in sub-Saharan Africa and North America, in that those of sub-Saharan Africa further reduce the risk of severe COVID-19 disease whereas those of North America increase susceptibility to severe disease in African Americans.

The Nature of the Disease

Severe acute respiratory syndrome coronavirus 2 (SARS-CoV-2) has a marked tropism for the biliary tract: it damages the bile ducts and hepatocytes and can lead to liver decompensation, cirrhosis, and sepsis. Liver damage in turn is linked to thinning and leaky blood vessels and to lung, heart, and brain damage. The author and colleagues have proposed that SARS-CoV-2-associated liver damage induces the protean manifestations of COVID-19 disease due to the spillage of stored retinyl esters into the circulation in toxic concentrations, and the features of the disease represent an endogenous form of hypervitaminosis A.[10,11] Anything that causes or contributes to liver damage and to increasing concentrations of vitamin A would therefore be expected to worsen the outcome of COVID-19 disease. Indeed, chronic liver disease is significantly associated with poor clinical outcomes of the disease.[12]

Apparently contrary to this hypothesis, serum retinol concentrations are markedly reduced in patients with severe COVID-19.[13] Such findings have been interpreted as indicating vitamin A deficiency and led to recommendations for vitamin A supplementation.[14, 15] Low retinol levels in patients with COVID-19 could instead be due to liver damage and to impaired mobilization and secretion,[16] but in association with the spillage of stored retinyl esters into the circulation in toxic concentrations; that is, hypervitaminosis A, the exactly opposite state. Vitamin A toxicity in adults is currently defined as a ratio of serum retinyl to total vitamin A (esters plus retinol) >10%.[17] To date, neither retinyl esters nor retinoic acid concentrations and expression have been measured in patients with COVID-19 disease, and the vitamin A toxicity hypothesis remains untested.

Evolutionary Adaptations to the Ancestral Environment

The prevailing view of disparities in health care access, quality, and health outcomes affecting African Americans is that they are due to social and economic factors that are historically rooted in structural racism and discrimination.[18-21] Less well known is that people of West Central African descent are also at reduced risk of death from other diseases, notably malaria, dengue hemorrhagic fever, yellow fever, and nonalcoholic fatty liver disease.[22-25]

These mostly infectious diseases are prevalent in West Central Africa, suggesting genetic links between the natural environment and endemic vector-borne diseases. Here it is suggested that the overall health profile of people of West Central Africa and their descendants has resulted in part from protective physiological adaptations to potentially lethal endemic parasitic organisms, most notably *Plasmodium falciparum*, occurring over an evolutionary timescale. On the proposed theory, inherited physiological characteristics acquired over millennia from adaptations to endemic tropical diseases – including malaria, schistosomiasis, and onchocerciasis – render people of West Central African descent particularly sensitive to vitamin A as a toxin.

With regard to malaria, the parasites spend over a week in the human liver, where they selectively absorb vitamin A.[26] My hypothesis is that upon emerging from the liver packed with vitamin A, the merozoite-stage parasites use it as a cell membrane destabilizer to invade and reproduce in the red blood cells. As the damaged RBCs begin to die, the stored vitamin A is released into the circulation, causing the signs and symptoms of malaria as an endogenous form of hypervitaminosis A.[27] This hypothesis was tested in patients with *P. vivax* in Korea and showed, as expected, that serum retinol levels were significantly lower but retinoic acid concentrations were significantly increased compared to those of controls.[28]

The proposed evolutionary adaptations were 1) sequestering vitamin A away from the liver, where it is mainly stored, to other organs, to reduce its accessibility to the invaders; and 2) slowing the metabolism and catabolism of vitamin A, causing it to accumulate to subtoxic concentrations, thereby weakening the parasite and serving to reduce the risk of severe disease. These adaptations may have enhanced survival from *P. falciparum* in the original African environment, as well as from COVID-19 in the 2019-2022 pandemic, but have increased susceptibility to COVID-19 and chronic inflammatory diseases related to vitamin A in the environment of North America.[29]

The Impact of Different Microbial and Dietary Environments in sub-Saharan Africa and North America

The potential toxicity of vitamin A from its accumulation is reduced by at least two factors in the West Central African environment. The first factor is exposure to other tropical parasitic organisms, including *Schistosoma*, which lower *P. falciparum* densities and reduce the severity of malarial infection[29] by absorbing vitamin A from the host and thereby helping to balance the potential toxicity of vitamin A. The second factor is the traditional West Central African diet,[30] which is low in preformed vitamin A and high in vitamin A-absorbing fiber. In sum, evolutionary adaptations to the risk of death from malaria, coupled with the existing microbial and dietary environment of West Central Africa, may have helped to reduce the risk of severe malaria and of COVID-19, both of which involve the liver and are hypothesized to involve an endogenous form of hypervitaminosis A in disease pathogenesis; in malaria via the death of infected red blood cells filled with retinoic acid, and in COVID-19 via the release of stored vitamin A from the damaged liver into the circulation in toxic concentrations.

In contrast, the North American environment is characterized by the relative absence of vitamin A-absorbing parasites and by a dairy-based, vitamin A-rich diet, derived from the historic dependence of people of northern European ancestry on grazing animals. The proposed adaptations and environmental exposures cause vitamin A to accumulate, rendering people of West Central African descent in North America particularly sensitive to vitamin A as a cellular toxin, and at greater risk of the same chronic inflammatory diseases that affect European Americans. The increased concentration of vitamin A in organs outside the liver, together with its overall accumulation, are proposed to explain the susceptibility of African Americans to organ-specific diseases that were once rare in the original environment and are increasingly linked to vitamin A toxicity via mitochondrial dysfunction and apoptosis.[31]

Conclusions

People of West Central African descent may be more sensitive to vitamin A as a toxin than those of northern European descent, and disparities related to COVID-19 and chronic inflammatory diseases are proposed to be due in part to excess expression of the same retinoid-related mechanisms responsible for these diseases in general. SARS-CoV-2 targets and damages the liver and is theorized to lead to the release of stored retinoids into the circulation in toxic concentrations, causing the signs and symptoms of the disease. This could explain the fact that pre-existing liver disease increases the risk of severe COVID-19. The vitamin A toxicity hypothesis suggests that adoption of traditional or modified West Central African-style diets, which are low in preformed vitamin A and high in vitamin A-absorbing fiber, could help to prevent and treat COVID-19 as well as chronic inflammatory diseases involving vitamin A. Subject to testing, such diets could serve as a population-based strategy for maintaining overall health and increasing longevity.

References

1. Ndugga N, Hill L, Artiga S. COVID-19 Cases and Deaths, Vaccinations, and Treatments by Race/Ethnicity as of Fall 2022 https://www.kff.org/racial-equity-and-health-policy/issue-brief/covid-19-cases-and-deaths-vaccinations-and-treatments-by-race-ethnicity-as-of-fall-2022.
2. Parpia AS, Martinez I, El-Sayed AM et al. Racial disparities in COVID-19 mortality across Michigan, United States. EClinical Medicine 2021 Feb 26;33:100761. doi: 10.1016/j.eclinm.2021.100761.

3. Nolen S. Trying to Solve a Covid Mystery: Africa's Low Death Rates. New York Times, Global Health. March 23, 2022. https://www.nytimes.com/2022/03/23/health/covid-africa-deaths.html.
4. Soy A. Coronavirus in Africa: Five reasons why Covid-19 has been less deadly than elsewhere. UNICEF Oct. 9, 2020.
5. Ezeh A, Silverman M, Strange S. Why has Covid-19 had less of an impact in Africa? Quartz, Aug. 23, 2021. https://qz.com/africa/2049407/why-has-covid-19-had-less-of-an-impact-in-africa (Accessed February 11, 2023).
6. Wamai R. What could explain the lower COVID-19 burden in Africa despite considerable circulation of the SARS-CoV-2 virus? Int J Envir and Public Health August 2021; 18(16): 8638.
7. Chen K, Kaplow L, Kemi Onabanjo, SunChen YS et al. A data-driven approach to addressing COVID-19 vaccine uptake in Africa. McKinsey Aug. 2, 2022. https://www.mckinsey.com/industries/healthcare-systems-and-services/our-insights/a-data-driven-approach-to-addressing-covid-19-vaccine-uptake-in-africa (Accessed February 11, 2023).
8. Lewis HC, Ware H, Whelan M, Subissi L et al. UNITY Studies Collaborator Group. SARS-CoV-2 infection in Africa: a systematic review and meta-analysis of standardised seroprevalence studies, from January 2020 to December 2021. BMJ Glob Health 2022 Aug;7(8):e008793. doi: 10.1136/bmjgh-2022-008793. PMID: 35998978; PMCID: PMC9402450.
9. WHO Africa. 07 April 2022. https://www.afro.who.int/news/over-two-thirds-africans-exposed-virus-which-causes-covid-19-who-study).
10. Mawson AR, Croft AM, Gonzalez-Fernandez F. Covid-19: how a virus is turning the world upside down. BMJ 2020;369:m1336. doi: https://doi.org/10.1136/bmj.m1336 (Published 03 April 2020).
11. Mawson AR, Croft AM, Gonzalez-Fernandez F. Liver damage and exposure to toxic concentrations of endogenous retinoids in the pathogenesis of COVID-19 disease: hypothesis. Viral Immunol 2021 Jul-Aug; 34(6):376-379. doi: 10.1089/vim.2020.0330.
12. Nagarajan R, Krishnamoorthy Y, Rajaa S, Hariharan VS. COVID-19 severity and mortality among chronic liver disease patients: A systematic review and meta-analysis. Prev Chronic Dis 2022; 19:210228. DOI: http://dx.doi.org/10.5888/pcd19.210228
13. Sarohan AR, Akelma H, Araç E, Aslan Ö, Cen O. Retinol depletion in COVID-19. Clin Nutr Open Sci 2022 Jun;43:85-94. doi: 10.1016/j.nutos.2022.05.007.

14. Stephensen C, Lietz, G. Vitamin A in resistance to and recovery from infection: Relevance to SARS-CoV2. Br J Nutrition 2021; 126(11):1663-1672. doi:10.1017/S0007114521000246.
15. Midha IK, Kumar N, Kumar A, Madan T. Mega doses of retinol: A possible immunomodulation in Covid-19 illness in resource-limited settings. Rev Med Virol 2021 Sep;31(5):1-14. doi: 10.1002/rmv.2204.
16. Olsen K, Suri DJ, Davis C, Sheftel J, Nishimoto K, Yamaoka Y, Toya Y, Welham NV, Tanumihardjo SA. Serum retinyl esters are positively correlated with analyzed total liver vitamin A reserves collected from US adults at time of death. Am J Clin Nutr 2018 Nov 1;108(5):997-1005. doi: 10.1093/ajcn/nqy190. PMID: 30475970; PMCID: PMC6692705.
17. Saeed A, Dullaart RPF, Schreuder TCMA, Blokzijl H, Faber KN. Disturbed Vitamin A Metabolism in Non-Alcoholic Fatty Liver Disease (NAFLD). Nutrients. 2017 Dec 29;10(1):29. doi: 10.3390/nu10010029. PMID: 29286303; PMCID: PMC5793257.
18. Institute of Medicine. Unequal Treatment: confronting racial and ethnic disparities in health care. Washington, DC: National Academies Press, 2002.
19. LaVeist TA, Isaac LA (eds.) Race, Ethnicity and Health: A Public Health Reader, Second Edition. Jossey-Bass, San Francisco, 2013.
20. Williams DR, Lawrence JA, Davis BA. Racism and health: evidence and needed research. Ann Rev Public Health 2019; 40(1):105-125.
21. Colen CG, Ramey DM, Cooksey C et al. Racial disparities in health among nonpoor African Americans and Hispanics: The role of acute and chronic discrimination. Soc Sci Med 2017. pii: S0277-9536(17)30290-3. doi: 10.1016/j.socscimed.2017.04.051.
22. Adu B, Dodoo D, Adukpo S, Gyan BA, Hedley PL, Goka B, et al. (2011) Polymorphisms in the RNASE3 Gene Are Associated with Susceptibility to Cerebral Malaria in Ghanaian Children. PLoS ONE 6(12): e29465. https://doi.org/10.1371/journal.pone.0029465
23. Blake LE, Garcia-Blancoa MA. Human genetic variation and yellow fever mortality during 19th century U.S. epidemics. mBio 2014; 5(3). e01253-14 https://doi.org/10.1128/mBio.01253-14
24. Gainor EM, Harris E, LaBeaud AD. Uncovering the Burden of Dengue in Africa: Considerations on Magnitude, Misdiagnosis, and Ancestry. Viruses. 2022 Jan 25;14(2):233. doi: 10.3390/v14020233. PMID: 35215827; PMCID: PMC8877195.
25. Samji NS, Snell PD, Singal AK et al. Racial Disparities in Diagnosis and Prognosis of Nonalcoholic Fatty Liver Disease. Clinical Liver Disease 2020; 16:66-72. https://doi.org/10.1002/cld.948

26. Mizuno Y, Kawazu SI, Kano S, Watanabe N et al. In-vitro uptake of vitamin A by Plasmodium falciparum. Annals of Tropical Medicine & Parasitology 2003; 97(3):237-243,
DOI: 10.1179/000349803235001723
27. Mawson AR. The pathogenesis of malaria: a new perspective. Pathog Glob Health. 2013 Apr;107(3):122-9.
doi: 10.1179/2047773213Y.0000000084.
28. Na J, Khan A, Kim JK, Wadood A, Choe YL, Walker DI, Jones DP, Lim CS, Park YH. Discovery of metabolic alterations in the serum of patients infected with Plasmodium spp. by high-resolution metabolomics. Metabolomics. 2019 Dec 23;16(1):9.
doi: 10.1007/s11306-019-1630-2. PMID: 31872321.
29. Mawson AR. Understanding health disparities affecting people of West Central African descent in the United States: An evolutionary perspective. Evolutionary Applications 202; 16:963–978.
https://doi.org/10.1111/eva.13549
30. Briand V, Watier L, Le Hesran JY, Garcia A, Cot M. Coinfection with Plasmodium falciparum and schistosoma haematobium: protective effect of schistosomiasis on malaria in Senegalese children? Am J Trop Med Hyg. 2005 Jun;72(6):702-7. PMID: 15964953.
31. African Heritage Diet. Oldways. https://oldwayspt.org/traditional-diets/african-heritage-diet#:~:text=In%20Central%20and%20Western%20Africa, kale%20and%20maize%20(cornmeal). (Accessed February 6, 2023).
32. de Oliveira MR. Vitamin A and retinoids as mitochondrial toxicants. Oxid Med Cell Longev 2015; 2015:140267. doi: 10.1155/2015/140267. Epub 2015 May 19. PMID: 26078802; PMCID: PMC4452429.

INDEX